STR@ESS
HOME

A Handbook of 40 Stressbusters for Housewives

STR@SS
HOME

A HANDBOOK OF 40 STRESSBUSTERS FOR HOUSEWIVES

Seema Gupta

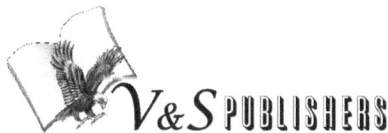

V&S PUBLISHERS

Published by:

V&S PUBLISHERS

F-2/16, Ansari Road, Daryaganj, New Delhi-110002
011-23240026, 011-23240027 • *Fax:* 011-23240028
Email: info@vspublishers.com • *Website:* www.vspublishers.com

Branch : Hyderabad
5-1-707/1, Brij Bhawan (Beside Central Bank of India Lane)
Bank Street, Koti, Hyderabad - 500 095
040-24737290
E-mail: vspublishershyd@gmail.com

Follow us on:

For any assistance sms **VSPUB** to **56161**

All books available at **www.vspublishers.com**

© **Copyright:** V&S PUBLISHERS
ISBN 978-93-813841-1-4
Edition 2013

Printed at : Param Offseters, Okhla, New Delhi-110020

Dedicated to.....

*All those housewives
who love to live
a stress free life*

Acknowledgements

I would like to take this opportunity to thank a few people who helped me make this dream a reality.

First of all, I must thank my mother-in-law, Mrs. Avdhesh Gupta who taught me the intricacies of life and value of relationships.

Besides the all round help and unfailing support extended to me by my husband, Mr. A.K. Gupta and my daughters, Aashima and Ameesha. I wish to acknowledge my sincere thanks to Mr. Ram Avtar Gupta, Managing Director of Pustak Mahal for his support and encouragement to me to author this book. Without his support and encouragement, this book would not have been possible.

I also extend my grateful thanks to Mr. S.K. Roy, Executive Editor of Pustak Mahal for his unfailing help and guidance. It is his faith in my abilities which enabled this book to see the light of the day.

—Seema Gupta

Contents

My Word

When I began my tryst with **Psychotherapy and Counselling**, I was amazed at the vast number of women suffering from personality disorders owing to the pressure mounting within them due to increasing stress.

Here I would particularly like to mention this case which is a perfect example of how stress accumulated over the years, can play havoc with not only a person's own life but with the lives of others associated too. There was this lady who had a teenaged daughter who was to write her class XIIth board exams that year. The lady wanted her daughter to be a doctor whereas the daughter was more keen on doing engineering. The girl was good at studies and had scored 87% in her Xth boards. While choosing her stream in class XIth, the girl wanted to opt for Maths and Computers in the Science stream while the mother insisted on her studying Biology. After much persuasion, the girl opted for Biology as well as Mathematics, (though she hated Biology), so that she could appear for the competitive examinations for both medical as well as engineering.

The mother, being a housewife, diverted all her energies to the girl and tried forcing her to give more attention to Biology. The girl, though, more keen on engineering, could not ignore her mother. The girl fared poorly in her exams in class XI, not only in Biology but in all the subjects. The mother was shattered. Having sensed that the mother was disappointed with her performance, the girl lost her self confi dence. She not only fared poorly in her XIIth boards, but could not clear any competitive test either. This was the last straw. The mother became depressed and went into a shell. When the mother came for counselling, she was reluctant to talk at first. As the sessions progressed, it was revealed that she came from a nuclear family where her parents were both successful doctors. She herself could not get into medical so she was trying to fulfil her unfulfilled ambitions through her daughter. She, herself being a lonely and sort of neglected child at home, showered extra love and attention on her daughter which in time turned into possessiveness. The lady also had a domineering husband, so she resented not having her own career. She was answerable to her husband for all the money she spent. That was the stress factor which triggered her to force her daughter to take up a lucrative career to have a solid financial background too. The lady, in her young age, had seen her doctor parents as a very compatible couple, so it was etched in her psyche that a doctor can have the best of both worlds.

After many counselling sessions, she came to terms with reality and when her daughter joined B.Tech. (Aeronautics), she was more than happy for her.

The fact, I am trying to emphasize here is that stress is a part of our lives, but we should not let it dominate us. Just like a diabetic may have an urge to eat sweets but he should refrain from it considering the ill effects of sugar on his health; similarly, we must learn to cope with the stress by identifying the stressors in daily life.

The following pages would give you an insight on **managing stress** through relaxation techniques, by adopting healthy habits, meditation and discovering happiness in your **present** rather than delving in the **past** or worrying about **the future**.

The five sets of questionnaire are given separately to help you in assessing your stress levels and to give you an insight on how well to cope with stress at all levels.

Here is wishing you a happy and stress free reading.

—**Seema Gupta**

Stress – The Silent Killer

'To me, the very essence of education is the concentration of mind and not the collection of facts.'

— Swami Vivekananda

'The real difficulty is always in ourselves, not in our surroundings.'

— Sri Aurobindo

During *Surya Namaskar*, each morning, when the bright sun rays touch my face gently, I feel light and relaxed. As the day progresses, the weight of emotions bogs me down and I wish for another ray of light from divinity to give me a fresh lease of life.

For a long time, I kept introspecting as to what makes us tense and unhappy. I ended up relating each day with the four phases of life. The early morning hours, when we are at our happiest and most relaxed, are like the carefree days of our childhood. As the day progresses, work mounts, expectations increase and there is a pressure to prove oneself – stress begins its journey through adolescence. By the time, our day progresses towards the post noon period, we are huffing and puffing to achieve our targets with tension mounting each second, quite like adulthood in life when we are working continuously without realizing how stressed out we are. Finally, it is time to close the shop. We are tired, stressed and devoid of energy. Our body and mind are craving for a break. So we call it a day – yes, the old age is creeping in.

But there have been times when we all feel very happy throughout the day. This clearly indicates that we have the power to conquer stress bodily, emotionally, intellectually and spiritually.

The first thing that comes to our mind is how do we defineSTRESS! Is stress a frown on our forehead or shaking of our hands in anger?

Stress is not something that affects us from outside. It is not an acquired trait by some unfortunate individuals. Stress is an integral part of the physical and mental system in all of us. We have inherited it during the course of evolution as a vital ingredient for normal functioning of the body. **Stress can be defined as a form of tension in our body or mind for which there is no release.**

Stress helps us in our survival on a sustained basis. But unchecked and uncontrolled stress can cause more harm to us than help. It can act as a **silent killer** and can erode our immune system leaving us vulnerable to many physical, psychological and personality disorders.

In simple words, stress is something that happens to our body whenever we are faced with a challenging situation.

The world witnessed stress for the first time when life itself originated on earth. Remember, the Darwin's theory of **'Survival of the Fittest'**. For people in those times also, it would have been equally stressful having to fight for each morsel, an inch of space or merely trying to survive. Stress always was and still is vital for our survival.

Does that mean stress is not bad for us? Exactly, that's the point!... In fact, stress is a motivating factor in our lives. However, the continuous and accumulating stress is detrimental to our mental and physical well being. We need to tame our feelings. Its optimum level provides the best opportunities to surging talents, energies and happiness.

We need not make any effort to get rid of stress because it would be futile. What we need to understand is that stress should be positive and conducive to our survival.

Social Norms

When I was a child, once I went to my grandmother's house. She lived in a village. One day, we heard the loud banging of thali (plate) in a nearby house. I asked my grandmother as to what this commotion was all about. She told me that their neighbour has been blessed with a son. When I asked her, how could she be so sure that it is a son when she had not even seen the baby, she laughed and said, "only a son's birth can bring such happiness to the family which they express by striking a thali. A girl's birth would have gone unnoticed." I was too young to understand the real impact of her words then. I just mingled with everyone there and joined in their rejoicing on having got a heir. Now after three decades, when I look back, it hurts me to see that not much has changed for women in our society. They are still the weaker sex and are still being treated unfairly.

Society has set certain norms for women which they are expected to abide by. You must have heard of the Hindi movie, 'Fire' made by Deepa Mehta. It was about two women who turned into lesbians. Now this movie certainly defied all norms of the Indian society and Deepa Mehta received flak from all sections of the society. She had to bear their wrath so much so that she could not make the next three films in her much talked about series.

There is a rebel hidden within each woman, which tries to free her from all shackles, but her conditioning over the years forces her to keep a low profile. There may be a few exceptions to the rule, but by and large, women prefer to stick to the norms of the society. However, somewhere deep inside them lies buried a desire to be able to live their life as they wish. This suppressed desire turns into stress and harms her emotionally, mentally as well as physically.

There was a girl, I knew, who got married at a very young age. In her in-laws' family, it was a custom to change the girl's name after marriage. The same was followed with her. She was also given a new name. Now by sheer chance or luck, in her maternal home, there was a servant by the same name. The girl could not protest as she was taught to be submissive. Initially, no one said anything about this. Later on, when everyone got to know of this fact, they started teasing her. But it was very late by then. The new name stuck to her, so did the stigma. This comparison kept burning within her and this sweet natured girl turned into an irritable, short-tempered woman.

Women are a less privileged group. This has been accepted offi cially by the Government authorities also when they decided to allot a special quota for women in all spheres of life. Women are called **the weaker sex** because they are physically not as strong as men. But that does not make them any less important than men. Consider any fi eld, any sphere of life and you will see that women have excelled by virtue of their natural talent. All they need is some support and help from their loved ones. When it is denied then their desires and their hopes die within their heart. Since they are not able to express these feelings, they feel suffocated within themselves. These feelings when held back for long, give rise to stress. Some spend an entire lifetime with these stressors playing havoc with their lives. They feel helpless and resigned to fate in the manner of a sacrifi cial lamb. Various symptoms of stress bog them down as they are unable to do anything because of the pressures of the society on them.

Stress Management – 40 Tips

Outer circumstances and events do not create stress. It is our response to them which creates stress.

— Swami Satyanand

We all agree that stress is an integral part of our lives. A certain degree of stress is actually good for our growth. As excess of anything is harmful, similarly, excessive stress is also bad for us. Technically, whenever we perceive any physical or psychological threat, we come under the grip of stress. If I put it in a layman's language, it means that whenever our mind feels uneasy, restless, disturbed, agitated, tense or strained, we are said to be under stress. Then what is the stress free state of mind? When our mind is cheerful, feeling light, easy, calm and quiet, we are said to be in a relaxed state – this is the stress free state of mind. This is the state we enjoy and try to achieve it all the time. Once achieved, we long for it to last forever. But the irony of the matter is that while we try to cling to the relaxed state of mind, we come under so much stress in the process that we inadvertently put the stress back into our lives.

Strangely, this time, the cause for this stress is nothing else but our desire to be stress free. So while we know what stress is, what the stressors are and what are their repercussions, the most important thing in combating stress is **Stress Management**.

In this book, we shall take a look at the stressors in the life of an Indian housewife who has devoted her life to her husband, family and home. She is the homemaker.

There is a special conditioning of the traditional Indian woman who is a homemaker. She has been taught from the cradle onward to take life as it comes. There are rules and restrictions for her which she is not supposed to break but follow them blindly. While it is impossible to enumerate and list various prejudices, it is important to know that these ingrained notions add tremendously to the stress levels of these women. Many a times, these innocent victims are not even aware that they are living under stress because they are conditioned to accept it as a part of their life. They are called upon frequently to fall back on their so called resources of will power but all this leads to stress arousal.

Let's take a look at the stressors, a housewife faces in her daily life and how she copes with them.

Complexes

Emperor Akbar admired the wittiness of Birbal. He thought Birbal was so wise because he was a Brahmin. Emperor then decided to convert himself into a Hindu Brahmin. Birbal tried to dissuade him but to no avail. So Birbal escorted the emperor, looking for a holy man who could convert him into a Brahmin there. Akbar saw a man scrubbing a donkey. The man explained, "I am changing my donkey into a horse. A holy man said that if I stood by the river and scrubbed it hard it would turn into a horse." Akbar realised his folly and promised Birbal to change himself and not the religion. He will act and become a better man. Managing yourself is very important before you manage anyone else. SWOT analysis helps in doing this to a great extent.

Strengths, Weaknesses, Opportunities and Threats

- ♦ **Strengthening** wisdom, intelligence, patience, character.
- ♦ Controlling **Weaknesses** like anger, jealousy, arrogance.
- ♦ Grabbing **Opportunities** of good communication and knowledge.
- ♦ Facing the **Threats** of bad health, poor relations and low esteem.

Food on Other's Platter

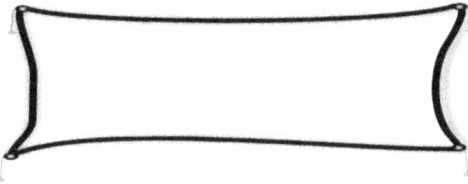

Power and money attract everyone. As you pass through different phases in life, your priorities also change. Initially you may choose to settle down to a quiet life of marital bliss rather than getting into the rut of a nine to five job.

But as the initial euphoria of marriage settles down, you may seek the change and start thinking, 'Why can't I be a career woman like her?' And so on.....

Rubina rushed to the balcony to say goodbye to her husband who was leaving for office. She was aghast to find him looking at someone else rather than waving at her. She followed his gaze and was shocked to find him looking appreciatively at Mrs. Nahata, who, too, was rushing off to office.

An array of emotions, most of it envy, rushed through her body. Why can't I be in her place? Why am I cooped up in this flat rushing through housework each day without any respite while she and her kind enjoy life in the office? The feeling stayed with her all day long, day after day, making her tense and irritable.

Every situation has two sides. It is up to us how we perceive that situation.

Positive Aspects

♦ By being a housewife, you can adjust your chores according to your own convenience. You do not have to rush through jobs.

♦ You can cook nutritious food for your family and feed them in a relaxed manner.

♦ Children grow up in the security of your love and protection.

♦ Your house would always be clean and tidy making you feel like a proud owner.

Negative Aspects

♦ What you lose by not being a working woman depends on your own perspective.

♦ Yes, by working in an office away from home, you may be able to escape the monotony of a routine life. But what is the guarantee that after a point of time, going to office itself will not turn into a monotony for you!

♦ So why get stressed over something in which you have nothing to gain, anyway.

Just because you are not able to step into other person's shoes, you should not become tense and stressed. Everything has its negative and positive aspects. Weigh your options, keeping your priorities in mind.

If you are so keen on doing a job, you may take up a part-time job or turn freelancer, so that you can devote time to your family and have creative satisfaction too. Once your children grow up, you can take up a full-time job.

Consider all the positive aspects of being a housewife and tell us the truth. Do you still wish to get into that hectic schedule of constant running and rushing into things? Won't you rather enjoy life at your own pace? You are the boss in your house. So relish what has been served on your platter.

Remember, food on the other table always looks tempting but it turns sour as soon as it is placed on your table.

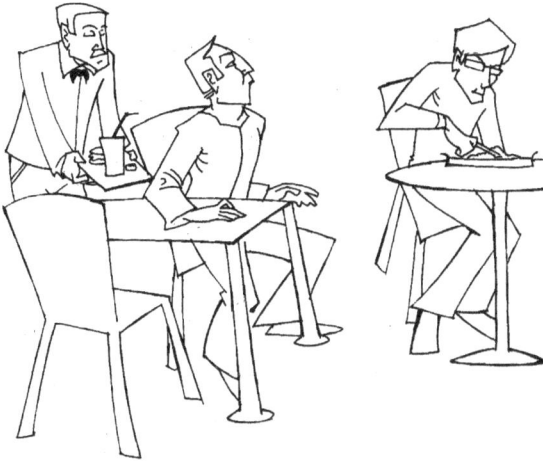

TIP OF THE DAY

Smile all day at everything and everyone that deserves a smile and see how many smiles you get back.

Chic and Smart

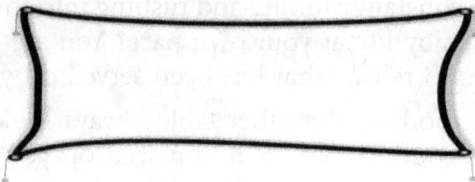

Every man wants his wife to look chic and smart. He may wear a combination of a red shirt and green pants and look like an oversized parrot, but he would like to hold a beautiful, well-maintained, well dressed woman by his side. So be it. It's for your own good.

Rita enviously looked at the ladies who would be impeccably dressed early in the morning, all ready to go to office. Rita was a housewife, so she found no reason to get ready early in the morning with various mundane chores waiting for her. By the time, she would be free, it's time for the kids to come back from school, so she would hastily take a bath and change into something comfortable, which was certainly not trendy. Within her heart, she nurtured a secret desire to look as smart as the working women. She wanted to look chic and smart, but how? Slowly this desire began to take over and she felt the stress of it in her life.

It is a general assumption that women who work in offices always look smarter than a housewife who is always seen in shabby and stained clothes. If a working woman looks chic and smart, it is because she has to go out of the house. Don't you also dress up smartly when you go out. Home is your working area. Since you are your own boss, you can choose to dress as you want. So if you feel like, you can dress up well even at home. After finishing the daily chores, wear ironed clothes, put on light makeup and relax. You will fi nd yourself feeling light and elated. A fresh and smart look is not only pleasing to others but it gives you also a feeling of satisfaction.

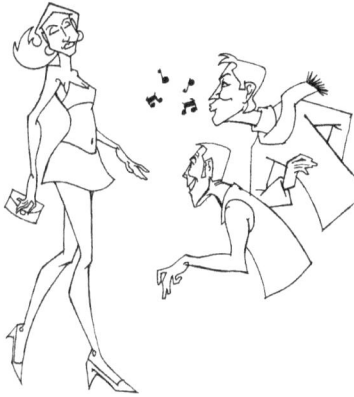

Getting dressed and visiting the nearby market will certainly lift your spirits. You need not dress like a beauty queen, but dressing up in a crisp cotton or silk saree will make you feel good and you will experience a confi dence you had never known before. Stay like this till your husband and kids come back and bask in the appreciative glances they throw at you.

TIP OF THE DAY

After getting all dressed up, choose your favourite fruit juice and sip it slowly while sitting in your favourite place and reading your favourite book. Feel the renewed energy seep through your body. These ten minutes will be the best part of your day.

B
U
S
T
E
R
3

Talent Search

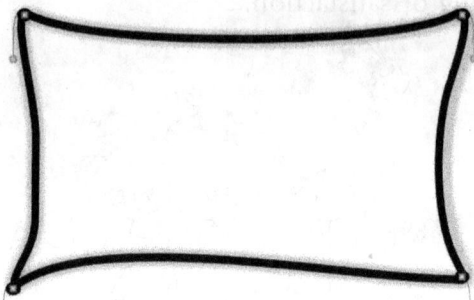

In our society, much emphasis is put on the beauty and complexion of a girl. A fair skinned girl is considered to be beautiful even if her features are not so appealing. Talent takes a back seat when it is compared to beauty.

Ranjana and Sunita are married to two brothers. Ranjana is fair complexioned whereas Sunita is dark complexioned as compared to Ranjana. Sunita is very talented. She has a sweet voice and sings beautifully. Although everyone in the family appreciates her talent, but when it comes to beauty, Ranjana takes an upper hand.

This stresses Sunita as she feels suffocated in Ranjana's presence, for the fear of comparison by other people.

When God created us, he gifted each one of us with an individual talent. If you overcome your feeling of guilt and give yourself a fresh beginning, you will find all your tensions evaporating.

Have you ever tried to look within yourself, search for that extra talent which will give you a different dimension in other people's eyes?

Feeling stressed over petty issues like complexion, beauty, texture of skin, etc., will not take you anywhere. Look for the real talent within you and search for the right avenues. You can polish your talent by practice and soon you will find everyone appreciating it.

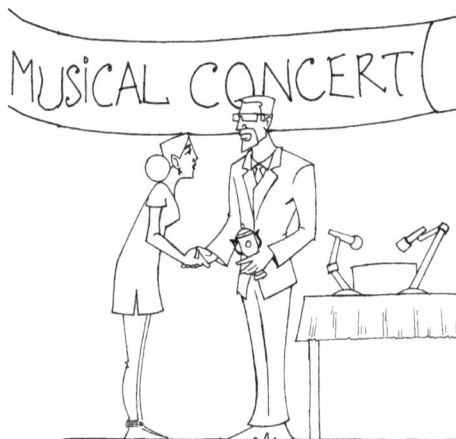

Learn to accept yourself as you are. Appreciate what is good in others, but not at the cost of your self esteem. You are what you want to be. So learn to be happy and count your blessings.

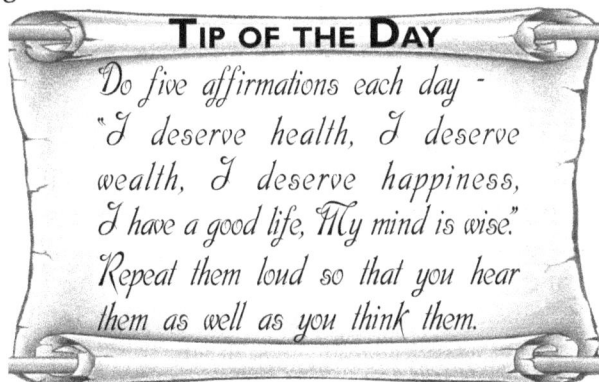

TIP OF THE DAY

Do five affirmations each day - "I deserve health, I deserve wealth, I deserve happiness, I have a good life, My mind is wise." Repeat them loud so that you hear them as well as you think them.

Height of Achievement

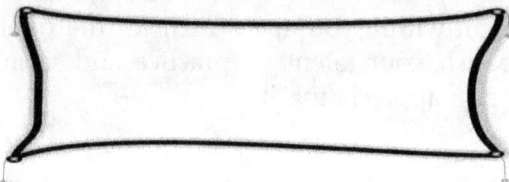

What have I achieved? What are my accomplishments after giving the best years of my life to this house?

... Are you constantly bothered by such questions? Living in the background while all the limelight is hogged by your husband or other members of the family, can be tiresome.

Mona was a computer engineer. Soon after she completed her studies, she got married. In due course of time, she had two children and soon, she was lost in the daily grind of cooking, looking after the home, kids and other mundane jobs. As the children grew up and started going to school, she found more time in hand. She started feeling a void within herself. She felt as if she had wasted half her life and now whatever is left will also go down the drain. She could not pinpoint a single thing which she could call her own achievement or anything that would give her sense of accomplishment.

In this life, we enjoy many comforts which we do not give much attention to. We are fortunate in having all our basic needs fulfi lled. We have all material comforts, a good family to share our joys and sorrows, neighbours to fulfi l our social needs, and good health. By looking after the home and children, a housewife is doing her duty. If her family is well nurtured, if her children are brought up well, is this any less achievement? Basically, the feeling of achievement is a state of mind. You may feel exhilarated at the first step taken by your child because it is an achievement too. Brooding over something which is illusive is pointless.

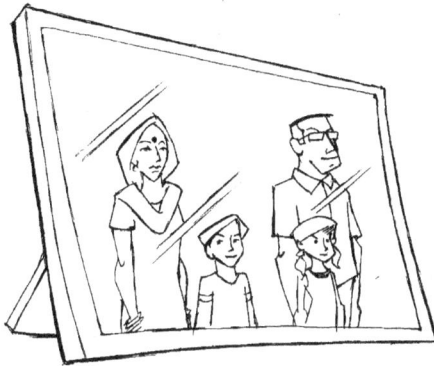

Learn to count your blessings. You are in no way inferior to others. It's only their way of living life which makes them different from you. So naturally, their achievements will be different from yours. Why bother to compare yourself with others.

TIP OF THE DAY

Challenge your comfort zone and see how alive you feel once you have achieved something you never dreamed was possible. A few options are :

Take a parachute jump

Touch a spider

Try a bungee jump

... The list may go on....

Fear of the Unknown

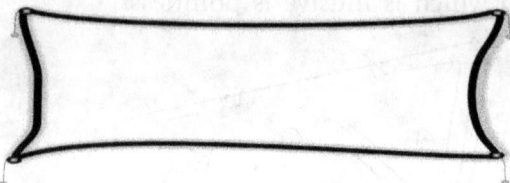

No two emotions are alike. If we are happy, we will be sad too. If we laugh, soon we will cry. So if we fear certain things in this world then we are also brave enough to face some bravely.

Trisha has a problem. Her husband is very popular with the ladies. He has enough compliments to shower upon them. He has interesting stories, jokes and anecdotes to share with them. Though he is an easy going guy, he is not loose on morals. Trisha has never caught her husband cheating on her, but his popularity seems to give her complex and a fear of the unknown.

If you are not sure of something then it is better to give it the benefit of doubt. Why fear for something which may not exist at all, except in your imagination? You should in fact be proud of your husband if he is popular.

Revel in the attention bestowed upon your husband and feel proud of it.

Remember, he may be friendly with other women, but you are the stabilizing factor in his life. He will never go astray, so long as you keep the reins tight and not give him

a chance to brood and go astray. So do not nag or fight.
Love him for what he is – a good natured human being.

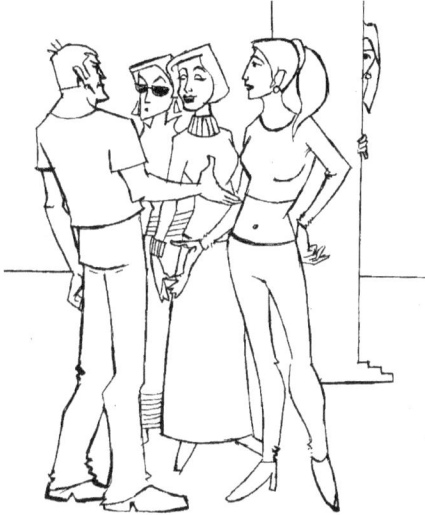

If the situation was reversed, and you were the one hogging
all the limelight, do you think you would leave your husband
for a few moments of fun – a revolting thought, isn't it? So
rest assured, nor would he.

TIP OF THE DAY

Cut on caffaine, sugar and refined food for a week. Eat only natural food and feel your spirits rise.

Stress in Joint Families

One day Akbar asked Birbal, "Tell me the difference between truth and falsehood in two words. Birbal said, "Four fi ngers." "Four fi ngers?" asked the Emperor, perplexed. "Your Majesty, what you see with your own eyes is the truth, but what you heard may not be true. The distance between one's eyes and one's ears is about four fi ngers, Your Majesty." said Birbal, grinning.

You see in others only what is in yourself.

You can't see faults in others unless the same faults exist in your.

The world is a laboratory where we conduct various types of experiments to learn various things and we ourselves are also tested off and on by facing various trials.

Unless you are ready to accept responsibility for the condition in which you are, there is very little that can be done to change that condition.

The best way to keep yourself happy is to ensure that others are happy.

Pressure Gauge

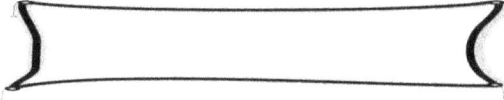

Every young girl dreams of a family where she is treated like a princess. She enters matrimony laced with rosy dreams. But real life is a far cry from her dreams. When reality hits her hard, all her dreams come crashing down.

When Sejal married, she had stars in her eyes. After the initial days of merry making were over, slowly the responsibilities started suffocating Sejal. She constantly complained to her husband that he never takes her out and doesn't bring her gifts often. They lived in a joint family so their house was always fl ooded with relatives. This would put an extra burden on Sejal. Sejal hated every moment doing house hold chores. But expectations from her in-laws made her slog the whole day long. She would crib and carry on with her work with a sullen face.

Life is ever changing. Remember the time you were young. The way everyone cuddled you and coochie-cooed you then, is not done once you grow up. You assume different dimensions in various relationships and they keep on changing with time. There was a time when your mother would feed you, but as you grow up, you start feeding yourself. You accepted this as a part of your life. Similarly, you should accept the fact that you are now married and have to fulfi l the responsibilities which come with it.

If the pressure in too much, it would be better to confide in someone who can make your in-laws understand your predicament. That person can be your sister-in-law, brother-in-law or your husband. Do not feel stressed as this is also a passing phase and you will soon get over it.

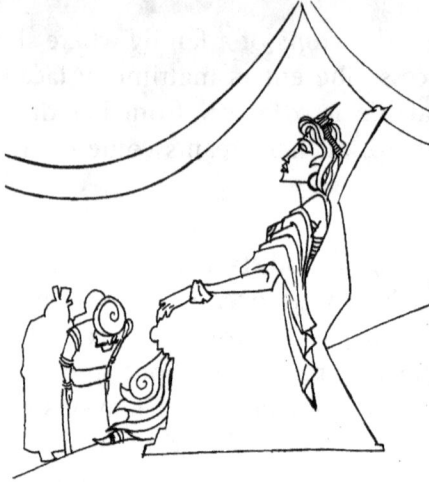

Enjoy the golden days of your life. Smile and everyone will smile with you. Soon, you will find many hands to help you and share your burden.

TIP OF THE DAY

When you feel stressed and want to shout, then go out to a lonely spot and yell and scream and stamp your feet. It does you good as well as to others – it stops you from thumping someone else.

Dowry – A Burning Issue

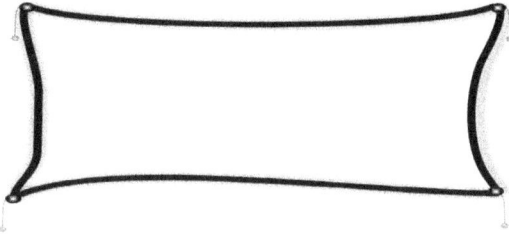

There was a time in India when dowry was a burning issue and many young brides became its victim. With the intervention of the Government and NGOs, new laws were passed and the Anti Dowry Bill was passed by the Parliament. Even after so many corrective measures, the fear of dowry still looms large in the mind of our brides which makes them feel insecure.

This reminds me of a funny incident which happened in our neighbourhood. When my neighbour, Mr. Khanna's only son got married, the bride came accompanied with all the dowry, as was asked by the Khannas. Except for demanding a few special items as dowry (as is the custom in their community), the Khannas, were basically nice people. But how was the new bride to judge this in a matter of a few days? After the couple came back from their honeymoon, the bride observed a bottle of kerosene oil kept in the kitchen with special care. On her own, the new bride decided that this bottle was kept there to burn her if she refused to bring any more dowry for them. One fine day, the television set she had brought as part of the dowry, broke down. The mother in-law was quite upset. Now the bride was very scared. She thought that she will be asked to replace it, which they did but only because all the papers were with the bride's father and the set was under guarantee. Unable to understand their view point, she refused to talk to her parents about the TV set at all and went into her room. As luck would have it, the electricity went off around one o' clock that night. This girl woke up when she heard some low voices coming from the kitchen. She could hear someone talking about kerosene and match box. Immediately, she came to the conclusion that her in-laws are planning to kill her by setting her on fire. She was under so much stress, that she could not think straight

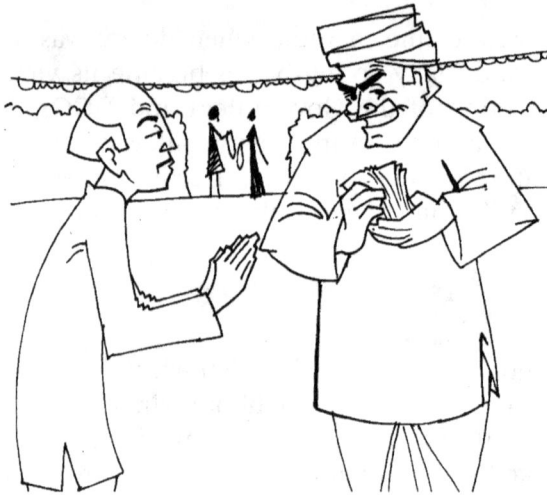

and instead of acting rationally, she just raised an alarm over nothing. The whole neighbourhood collected only to discover that the Khannas were actually trying to light a kerosene lamp. They were doing so in a hush hush manner so as not to disturb the young couple. Just imagine, what an embarrassing situation was created due to stress over an imaginary problem!

Does this give you an insight! However, if you feel that you are genuinely facing a threat, then do not delay things.

Take someone in confidence and take corrective measures immediately. Because it's your life.

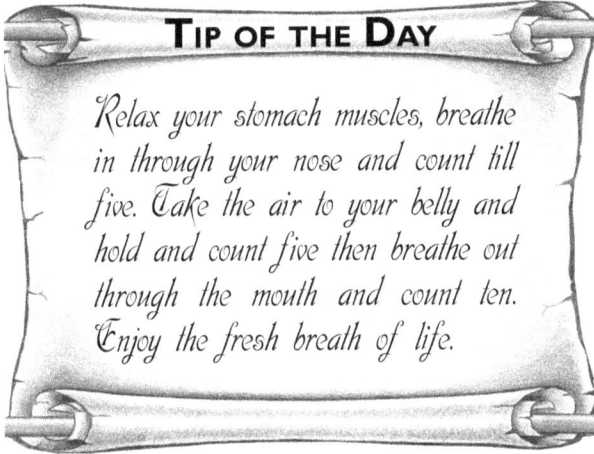

Daughter vs Daughter-in-law

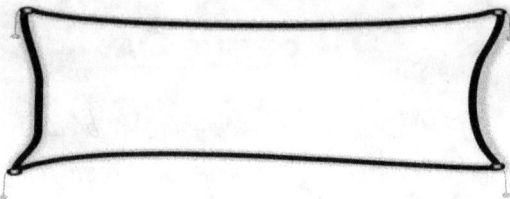

This is a very sensitive issue. A girl who spends twenty years of her life with her biological parents, is suddenly sent to a new house to spend the rest of her life amidst total strangers. However, much she may try, she cannot become the daughter of the house overnight.

Shweta and her husband's sister Mala were almost of the same age. When Shweta got married, Mala was in her fi nal year in college. Initially, the two of them became good friends. But as time passed, Shweta could distinctly feel the discrimination made by her in-laws between herself and her sister-in-law. Mala was allowed to wear all kinds of clothes, she could boogy with her friends, she could get up late, she need not cook proper meals in the kitchen and she was never ever spoken harshly by anyone. The treatment meted out to Shweta was totally in contrast. Shweta missed her parental home where she was he cynosure of all eyes. Shweta felt suffocated and her behaviour towards her new family started showing signs of rebel.

You have entered a new house where people are new, the rules are new. It takes time to adjust in a new place. Remember, you spent twenty years in that house which you considered your own. Now, how can you expect this house to become your own in just a matter of few days or weeks? Your sister-in-law has been here since birth, naturally, she feels the same as you feel towards your parental home. She is obviously getting the similar treatment which you were getting in your home before marriage. So have patience. Do not be hasty in making any decision. Each passing day will bring you closer to your new family.

As you become familiar with your new family, they too will begin to respond to you. No point in getting agitated over trivial matters and comparing yourself with your sister-in-law. Instead of competing, give her love and affection and rest assured, you will be reciprocated with similar feelings.

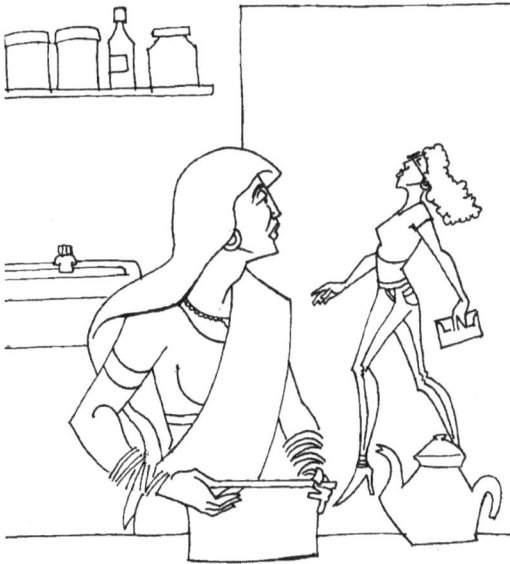

You may not be their daughter, but you are their daughter-in-law whom they have chosen with care, love and affection.

Why would they demean you? Put all the prejudices aside and love them like your own parents if you want to be their daughter. Soon, you will be more dearer to them than their own daughter.

TIP OF THE DAY

Be a dreamer. Allow yourself a dream time. Imagine yourself being carried away to a dreamland in your imagination. Return to this world refreshed and renewed. Remember, if you don't have dreams, they cannot come true.

Envy

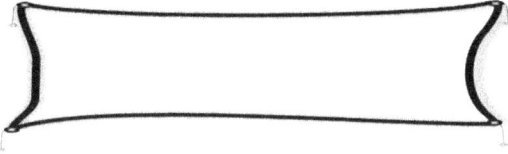

In a joint family, it is a common notion that wives of two brothers are always at loggerheads. Initially, they may live in harmony but as children arrive and the monotony of daily routine takes over, envy and tensions become the way of life.

Ruby and Sheena were good friends. They were married to two brothers. They lived in a joint family. Ruby was married to the elder brother. When Sheena came to the house as Ruby's younger sister-in-law, Ruby was ecstatic. Sheena also reciprocated her feelings. But as days passed by, various other emotions took over and the congeniality was replaced by envy and bickering between the two sisters-in-law. There was tension between them all the time. Fights among their children only added fuel to fi re. Life became hell in that house with tempers rising at the slightest pretext.

The elder sister-in-law has spent more time with the family than the younger sister-in-law so it is her duty to introduce the younger one to the new house. The younger sister-in- law, on the other hand, should give due respect to the elder one, as she is elder to her in age as well as in status. A little understanding and tact can go a long way. Fighting over children and their skirmishes is a foolish thing to do. Children forget and forgive more easily than elders. If you interfere in their matters, then you will only spoil your own relationships.

Who would like to live in a stressful environment? This will not only affect you but your children and other members of the family as well. Why should you envy each other? By living under the same roof, life can be very comfortable and enjoyable, but only if you maintain good relations.

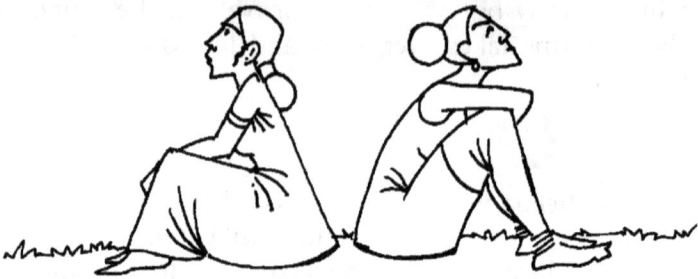

United we stand, divided we fall
Always remember this adage. Be there for each other in times of need. Instead of envy, spread love and trust and see your relationship blossom.

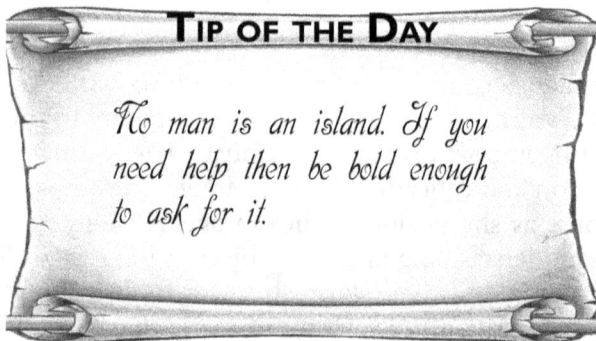

TIP OF THE DAY

No man is an island. If you need help then be bold enough to ask for it.

Interfering Relatives

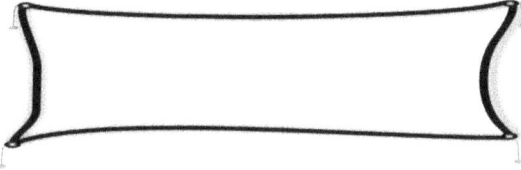

Life in a joint family is not a bed of roses if there are interfering relatives who dominate the thought process of the master or the lady of the house. If you are a working woman then you can escape these episodes by being away from home for better part of the day, but if you are a housewife, you have to bear the brunt stiffl y.

Raju and Meeta were married for two months. Meeta's mother-in-law Sharada, gave them lot of time together and did most of the work herself.

Life was peaceful until the day, Sharada's sister, Vimla came from Ahmedabad to spend a few days with the family. She was a very dominating person. She did not like the way her sister was handling her daughter-in-law. She influenced Sharada to bring the young bride to task and put all the household chores on her shoulders. Sharada relented and all hell broke loose for Meeta. She kept praying for the lady to leave.

Putting up a war in such situations will not take you anywhere. 'Endurance' is the keyword. Wait for a few days. Let the high tide pass. As the tempers cool down, you will fi nd it easier to get your point across.

If the relative is a guest in your house for a few days, then bear things with patience because soon it will be time for her to leave. Then you can go back to your normal routine. But if the person interfering is a member of your family then you need to talk things out as early as possible.

Do not feel so stressed. There is no problem in this world which has no solution. You can win anyone with love, affection and endurance. Getting stressed only makes matters worse.

Since you are a housewife, you will be interacting with them all day long. So instead of putting up a war front and facing them as your worst enemy, why not mingle with them and win their hearts? It may be tough, but not impossible.

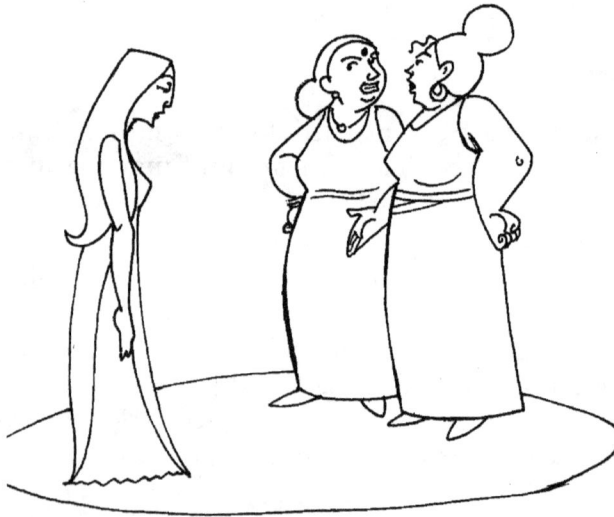

An old saying goes —

If you can't win them, join them.

This will be much better than living with the stress of having them as your critics forever.

TIP OF THE DAY

There is a Rose flower remedy for nearly every emotion. If you do not want to find out about all your emotions, then taking their rescue remedy will give you relief from many common emotional upsets. So discover the comfort in the essence of the Rose - calm is just a few drops away.

Stress in Nuclear Family

Emperor Akbar once asked Birbal, "Birbal is there anything that the sun and the moon cannot see?"

"Yes, Your Majesty, Darkness," came the prompt reply from Birbal.

In dwelling, live close to the ground,
In thinking, keep to the simple,
In confl ict, be fair and generous,
In governing, don't try to control,
In work, do what you enjoy,
In family life, be completely present.

If you can take care of things,
which are in your hands,
things which are not in your hands,
will be automatically taken care of.

No one was ever really taught by another.
Each one of us has to teach oneself in the long run.

Living Alone

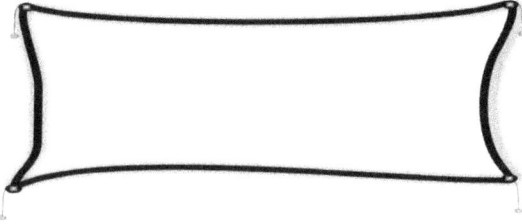

Living in a nuclear family is very different from living in a joint family. The concept of the nuclear family came into existence when India became global. The rural population started moving towards cities in search of better career prospects. Naturally, it was not possible for the whole family to move to a new place and abandon their roots altogether. So the immediate family such as the husband, wife and kids migrated. This new found freedom from the clutches of old family traditions gave them new wings and soon, the nuclear family became a big concept. Their stressors may be different from a joint family set up, but stress in a nuclear family cannot be totally ruled out.

Sheela migrated to Delhi from Jaipur, when her husband got a new job. She was very happy at having escaped the domineering mother-in-law and the never ending house hold chores in her in-laws' house. When her husband went to offi ce, she would fi nish all the chores quickly and relax. Sometimes, she would go for shopping. She felt relaxed and very happy. But the initial euphoria soon died and she started feeling very lonely in the house. She was used to living in a house full of people with their continuous chatter fi lling up every moment of the day. Here she hardly had anyone to talk to. There were no friendly neighbours and her hubby would be away for most part of the day. In the evening, he would be so tired that they hardly went out, except for the weekends. She felt that she lived only on weekends. Rest of the week stretched before her like a hot sandy road which she dreaded to tread. She started feeling tense as Monday approached.

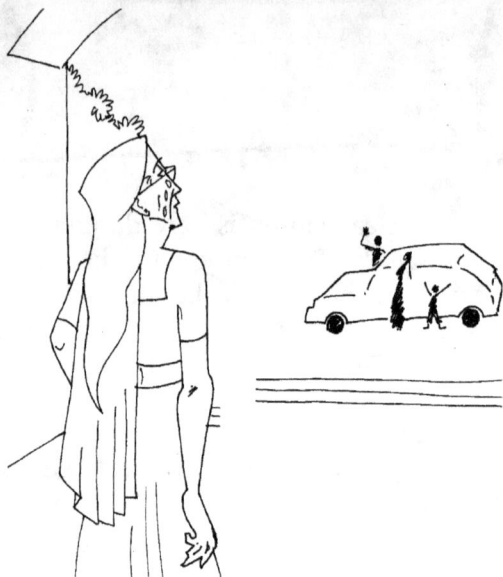

Living alone can be very taxing emotionally. You may enjoy the initial freedom but later on, when you are left in an empty house the whole day long, you may start dreading the long and lonely hours, especially, if you do not have a very friendly neighbourhood.

So the better way to deal with the situation is by making friends or keeping yourself occupied in various activities of your choice. You may join a hobby course which would not only enhance your skills but will also keep you occupied and give you an opportunity to meet people and make friends other than your neighbours.

The stress of having to while away the hours shows in your interaction with your husband when he comes back from work. You become more demanding. You need to go out more often because human beings are social beings and we need to interact with people. So come out of your shell. Big cities may sound aloof, but they also open many avenues for people and give them a chance to take part in group activities.

Remember, how you loathed the never ending housework in the joint family and how you treasure your privacy and independence here. Every situation has its own virtues and vices. So count your blessings and learn to adjust in every situation.

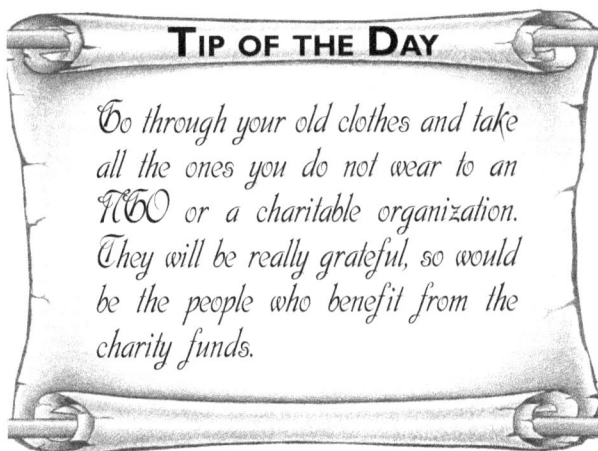

TIP OF THE DAY

Go through your old clothes and take all the ones you do not wear to an NGO or a charitable organization. They will be really grateful, so would be the people who benefit from the charity funds.

Resourceful

In a joint family, you pool in your resources and run the household. In this way, the burden does not fall on a single person's shoulders. But in a nuclear family, the entire responsibility of running the household falls on the only earning member of the family, since the housewife is not earning so her contribution in monetary terms is negligible.

Ritu's husband was an accounts offi cer in a private fi rm. But as the family grew and the cost of living went up, his income became insuffi cient in meeting the expenses. He picked up a part-time job. Life became very monotonous for Ritu as her husband became irritable with so much of work pressure. He would come home late and would be always tired. There was always shortage of money in the house and she had to be careful with the expenditure. Ritu was fond of going out and having fun but no luxuries were permitted in their existing budget. Ritu started feeling suffocated in this kind of atmosphere at home.

In today's times, this situation may rise in any household. With constant rise in infl ation, naturally, the husband has to work harder to make both ends meet. He may feel overworked and take out his stress on you. This gives rise to confl icts and the marital harmony may get disturbed. In such a situation, you are left with two options,either approach his parents or your parents and seek fi nancial help or cut down on your expenses. If he is working so hard to maintain a dignifi ed profi le then why can't you sacrifi ce some material comforts for him and share his burden?

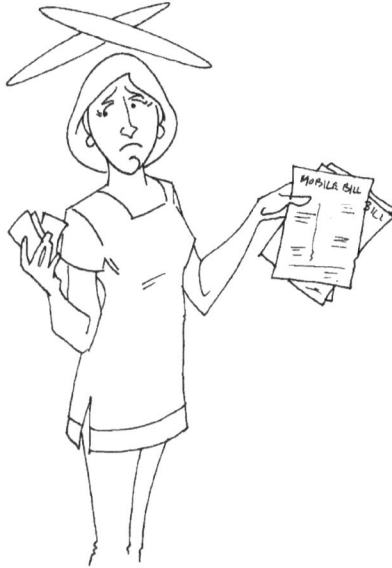

Your husband may be tired because of working overtime and coming late from offi ce. This is a stressful situation for a housewife who spends the entire day waiting for her husband. In return, she does not get even a loving smile from her tired husband on his return. Secondly, spending lavishly on luxury items would become diffi cult because you need to save for the rainy days too. All these factors together make a very stressful condition. But do not feel disheartened. Times do not always remain the same. On your part, you can also make an effort and try to organize something from home which can bring you fi nancial relief — like taking up a part time job or saving money on little things and by not being extravagant.

Stress is a part of our lives but letting it consume our lives completely will be pathetic. So find your happiness in small measures of everyday life and keep your cool. Remember if there is a problem, there has to be a solution nearby.

TIP OF THE DAY

Stimulate and nourish your mind by eating food for thought.

Choline in vegetables and eggs aid memory.

Inositol in grapefruit and cabbage nourishes brain cells.

Carbohydrates in pulses, rice and potatoes provide essential energy for our brain.

Mood Swings

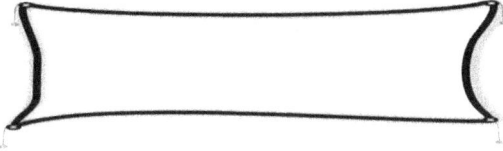

Your husband's mood swings can be easily controlled by a light scolding by his family members who are more prominent in a joint family. Since you are the only one around the house in a nuclear family, most of the time you become a victim of his wrath.

Ruchika's husband was very particular about keeping things in place whereas Ruchika herself was not such a perfectionist. She liked to keep things clean and tidy but not to the point when you cannot even relax on the sofa or enjoy a meal without having to worry about spilling the curry on the mat. But her husband was tidy to the tiniest detail. As evening approached, Ruchika would become a wreck as she did not know what might irk him and spoil the mood. The children would be huddled in their own room as their father's arrival came nearer. The same Ruchika who was a jolly and warm person when she lived in a joint family turned cold and withdrawn now. She felt helpless, not knowing whom to turn to for her husband's mood swings.

If the husband is a perfectionist, then it becomes a routine which can be very stressful to you. You may take your husband to be a heartless person who does not seem to care a bit for your feelings. Try to understand his predicament also.

He has lived so many years of his life with his perfection, so you cannot expect him to change overnight.

You can either make him see your point of view tactfully or take help of an elder person who has infl uence on him. The routine shoving of children in their room for the fear of spoiling the cushions or the seating arrangement is not good for their psyche. So take measure before it is too late.

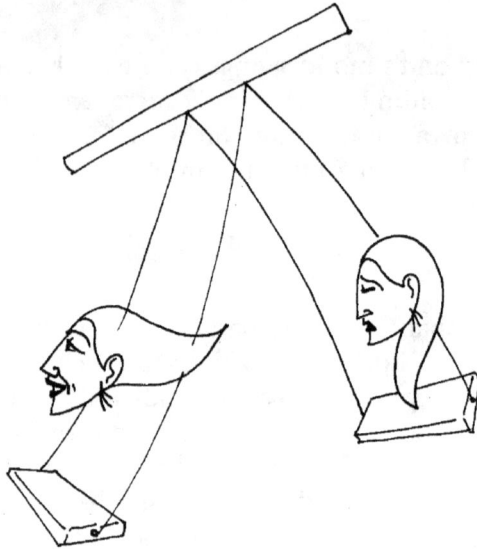

Don't look at your husband reproachfully. Everyone has his faults. If you were in his place, your mood swings would equally be stressful to the husband and kids because when they try to fi nd respite in the cool confi nes of a home, you would pounce on them for no fault of theirs.

Such situations arise only in nuclear families because there is no set code of conduct as is mostly found in joint families.

Before you get stressed, just imagine the kind of stress he must be facing on returning from office and while standing in front of the door. Being a perfectionist, his worst fears would be not to find things in place. Sympathize with him and do not be angry with him. Help him to get over his phobia.

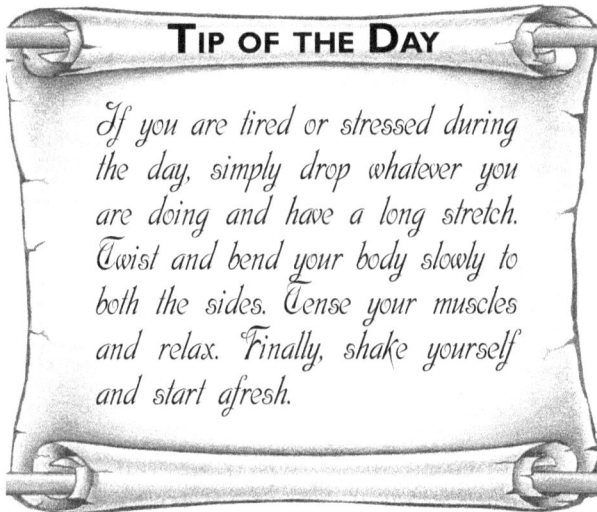

TIP OF THE DAY

If you are tired or stressed during the day, simply drop whatever you are doing and have a long stretch. Twist and bend your body slowly to both the sides. Tense your muscles and relax. Finally, shake yourself and start afresh.

Rejection

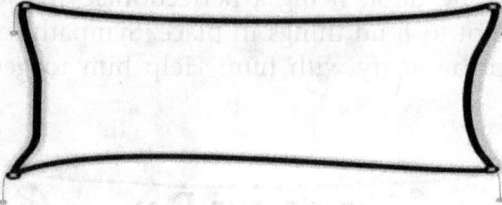

When you marry in a family, you want to become a part of that family. It takes efforts on both side to develop a compatible relationship. In most of the houses, if the daughter-in-law lives separately then she is rejected and considered as an outsider while the son remains to be a member of that family.

Shruti lived with her in-laws but she was constantly ridiculed for bringing insufficient dowry. She was trying her best to adjust with them when suddenly, her husband got transferred to a different city. It was a God sent solution for Shruti through which she could escape this stressful situation without much melodrama. They managed to set a separate home in the other city. But what irked Shruti most was the fact that her in-laws started treating her as an outsider. She was neither consulted in any family matter, nor was she apprised of any family functions, whereas her husband was posted of all the details. Shruti felt dejected and depressed. For no fault of hers, she was labelled an outsider.

The in-laws may not take kindly to a daughter-in-law who lives separately. This is an underlying stress because you lose a coveted position in the family. You may feel like an outsider when you are neither consulted nor told about the major decisions taken in the family. It is the time for you to take some steps. You can make some more efforts and improve your relations with the family members. It would be easier now, since you are living away from them and have already created your own space. Your efforts will not go unnoticed and sooner or later, either they will accept you or your husband will force them to accept you.

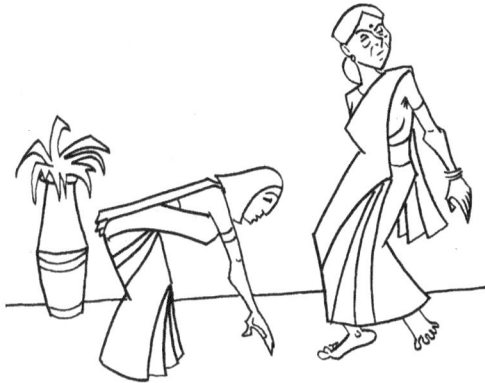

Your husband would never face such a problem because he is never blamed for the separation. It is always the daughter-in-law, who is not able to adjust and is thought to have taken the husband away from the cosy confines of his parental home. This unnecessary blame may make you tense. But say no to stress. Make efforts to carve your own place in this house.

If you wish to enjoy your freedom, do so in a subtle manner without hurting anyone. This will keep you stressfree and give you real happiness.

TIP OF THE DAY

If you are feeling very tensed, a cold shower leaves you feeling warm, invigorating and awake.

My Hands are Full

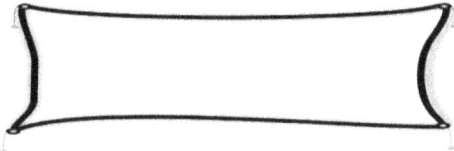

Bringing up small children is a big job. In a joint family, you get help from experienced people like your mother-in-law or your sister-in-law. But in a nuclear family, you may find yourself alone, nervous and fearful. Being inexperienced, you fear every move because you are not sure what is good for the baby. So you may either be running to the doctor for small things or calling up relatives to find out about the problems of infancy.

On top of that, you have to do the other household chores which you could easily escape in a joint family system. All this excessive work, running around and tension of bringing up the baby without any help keeps your stress levels very high and you start feeling fatigued very soon.

Sheela got separated from her in-laws when her daughter was barely two months old. She tried her best to manage everything but due to the burden of extra work, she became weak and tired. She was also neglecting her health. Her husband was not of much help either as he came back quite late from the office.

One day, as Sheela was out shopping, she felt giddy and fell down unconscious. The baby fell from her arms and started crying. There was a big commotion in the shop. Luckily, one of Sheela's neighbours spotted her and took her home. The baby was badly hurt and needed immediate medical attention. Sheela's husband was on tour. She had no choice but to call her in-laws and seek help.

Health is wealth. Excess work can be managed by hiring help in the form of maid if you have no one else to turn to. You must keep in mind that you can only look after your home and child if you are fi t and healthy. If you feel that you cannot manage alone then it is better to swallow your pride and patch up with your in-laws.

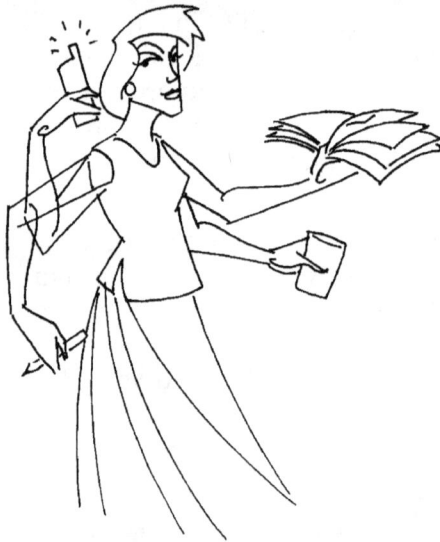

Just like this child is the apple of your eyes, similarly, your in-laws also love their grandchild. So do not shy away from them. Even if you are not living with them, maintain congenial relationships. They will extend all the help they can. This will certainly be much better than having to call them in an emergency and being labelled as a careless mother and a selfish daughter-in-law.

Parents are always there to help us. They would never disappoint their own children. Give them due respect and get lots of love from them in return.

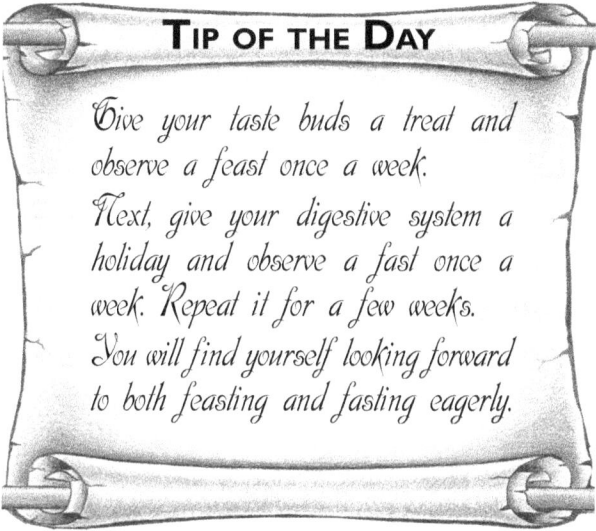

TIP OF THE DAY

Give your taste buds a treat and observe a feast once a week.

Next, give your digestive system a holiday and observe a fast once a week. Repeat it for a few weeks.

You will find yourself looking forward to both feasting and fasting eagerly.

Hubbies Howlers

One day Akbar was furious with his wife. In a fit of rage, he ordered his wife to leave his palace and go to her father's house. The queen was very upset. She called for Birbal. After narrating the entire episode, she asked for his advice. Birbal pacified her, "Do not worry. Such quarrels do occur in a family. Just do as I tell you and all will be well."

So the next day, the queen asked Emperor Akbar, "Your Majesty, I will do as you wish. But since I will not be seeing you again for the rest of my life, I would like to invite you to my palace for dinner tonight. Also please allow me to take with me my most precious possession that I may keep as your memoir."

That night, Akbar went to the queen's palace for dinner. She had prepared all his favourite dishes. At the end of the dinner, she offered him a glass of milk. The queen had added sleeping pills in the milk. As soon as Akbar finished the glass of milk, he fell asleep. The queen sent for Birbal.

Birbal arrived with a carriage. Akbar was put into the carriage and sent with the queen to her father's house. The next morning when Akbar woke up he looked around him puzzled. He felt strange. The room seemed unfamiliar. Then he saw the queen sitting at his bedside. She said, "Pardon me, my Lord. But you are in my father's house. If you remember, yesterday, you had granted me a wish to carry my most precious possession with me. So I have brought you along with me."

Akbar was touched by his wife's love. He realised his own folly and returned to the palace with the queen.

Love can overcome animosity.

Peaceful action against unreasonable opposition achieves the best results.

Silence is the hardest argument which can sometimes be offered to your opponent.

Made for Each Other

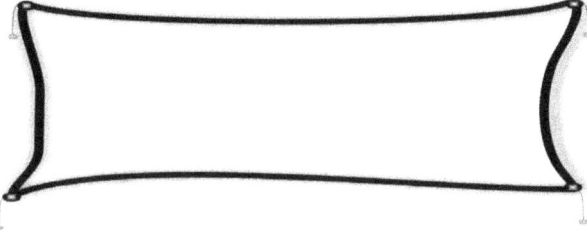

Love is the central element in a successful marriage. If that exists, all problems get sorted out. When you contemplate marriage, in your mind you have accepted that you want to build a relationship. The dreams, hopes and aspirations of two people are involved. When new relationships are formed, adjustments are imminent.

Sunita is married for ten years now. Her life has been sailing smoothly. She has a loving husband, two children and all material comforts. Yet she feels incomplete. She misses the love and attention showered by her husband in the initial years of marriage. She feels that her husband no longer finds her attractive and that is the reason why, he does not give her enough time. She cribs over it and often suffers from mood swings. Her husband tried to make her see reason but when nothing worked, he too gave up.

You expect the same treatment from your hubby as you received in the initial years of marriage but have you ever thought of giving him the similar treatment too? He is not complaining then why are you? As time passes, responsibilities increase and your time is divided. You still love each other but demonstrating this love takes a back seat. So do not feel stressed. Your husband is a sincere person. Your love is not lost, it has only matured over the years.

Cribbing or sitting in a corner and brooding for hours is not the best way to get your husband's attention. Put on your best clothes and cheerfully welcome him as he comes back home. Give him a surprise treat once in a while and revel in the glow that lights up in his eyes. Going for a stroll after dinner is a good idea. It boosts your health as well as the emotional equation. Plan a trip or an outing together. Leave the kids in the care of your parents or in-laws. You will come back refreshed.

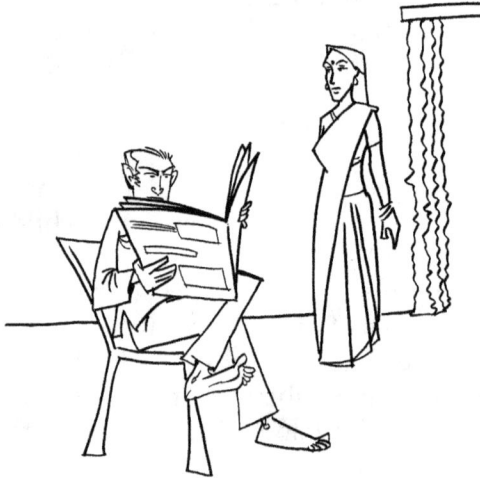

You were made for each other and that is why you are together. Do not let small events of life make you feel let down. Love is hiding behind the doors. Just knock and doors will open up for you.

Treat yourself to saunas and steam treatments. Sweat out toxins through steam and sauna. If you can do it together in the close proximity of your home, nothing like it.

Sharing the Burden

Most housewives depend upon their husbands for everything starting from financial support to doing teeny-weeny household chores. But this dependence acts like a handicap for them. They lean too much on their husbands. And at any point of time, the husband is not able to do the work, the dependent wife feels stressed.

Suchitra lived a very cushioned life. As she would never venture out of the house for shopping or other outside chores, her husband took over the responsibility. Even shopping for groceries, buying vegetables were all done by her husband on his way home. Suchitra only looked after the home. One fine day, her husband came home and informed her about his promotion and two months of training in Nagpur. She was devastated. How will she manage without him for two months? The thought of spending two months alone without anyone for support was a dreadful thought. The thought haunted her so much that she went into depression. Her husband tried to make her see the advantages of his training but the stress she was facing was beyond her control. Finally, her husband had to forego the promotion and cancel his training in Nagpur.

Is your dependence upon your husband costing him dear? Don't you think it is better to learn to be independent? In any case, being independent gives you a confidence. This confidence shows in your personality. All the housewives are well educated today. So why depend upon your husband for doing outside work? You can very well share his responsibilities. Be a helping hand, not a burden.

What makes you more stressed? A harassed, tired and short the tempered husband who does the outside work because you are unable to do it; or going out of the house and doing the jobs yourself. Choose your options carefully and see what benefi ts you more. Naturally, the latter is good for you as well as your hubby. At least, he won't snap at you now over trivial matters.

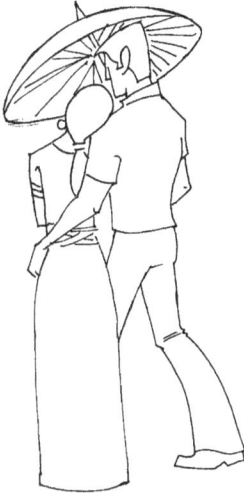

Earn your confi dence by being independent. Your husband will love you for the new glow on your face.

TIP OF THE DAY

Do some gardening. Get back to the earth and tend to natural, growing plants. Put something back into the Mother Earth and feel your spirits rise.

Budget Makers

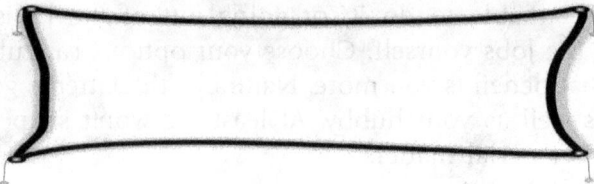

Since a housewife is not working, so naturally, she has no means of regular earning. Mostly the husband provides the money for household expenses. That is why, he is called the breadwinner of the house. But whatever amount the husband provides should be utilized wisely. You should be aware of your financial position and should be able to save for a rainy day.

Harish was the sole breadwinner of the family. His wife Suruchi never bothered to find out about his financial position. He too never indulged her into these matters. One day, as Harish was going to office, his car was crushed under a speeding truck. Harish survived but due to a spinal injury, he went into coma. He had to be operated soon. The operation required about three lakhs which had to be deposited as soon as possible. Suruchi was in a fix. She had no idea about their financial status. She did not even know where Harish kept his money, in which banks he had his accounts or from where she could borrow the money? Her husband was unconscious, so naturally, he was of no help in such a situation. She contacted her relatives and literally begged for help. When nothing came out, she sold her jewellery, mortgaged the house and deposited the required amount. After Harish recovered and came back home, he asked his wife as to how she managed to pay the money. He was aghast on being told that she had to mortgage the house for money. He took out the bank passbook and some bank FD's from his briefcase and showed her. Together they all contained more than five lakhs rupees. If only Suruchi knew about their financial position, she could have easily used that money instead of mortgaging the house. Now they had to pay a much bigger price to get their house back.

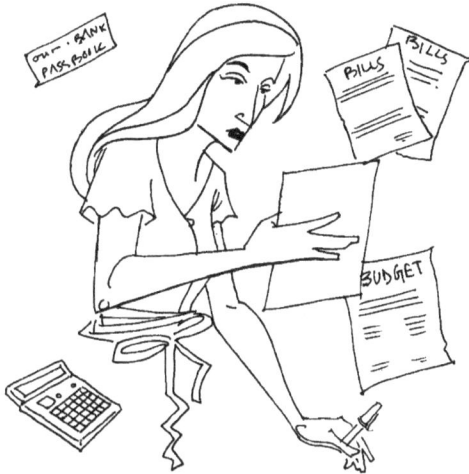

This is only one situation, we have taken up. There are many more everyday incidents, which point towards the fact, that money matters should be discussed among the husband and wife even if the wife is not working.

Dependence upon your husband can bring your stress levels high. Financial independence does not mean having to go out of the house to work. You can learn these things even by being a housewife. Learn about your finances. Go to the bank to deposit your cheques or withdraw the money. In this way, you will help yourself by being updated on your financial status.

If you have a keen interest in money, you may take tips from your husband and start investing in shares. Preparing a family budget together will also give you an insight on how to spend wisely. It will also help you get your priorities right.

Demonstrating your dependence on your husband in financial matters will only make you vulnerable and open to criticism. Money is important in life. So learn how to deal with it in a proper way.

TIP OF THE DAY

Do not live your life for other people all the time. Take out some time to try something that might not necessarily please everyone else but would give you great pleasure. Better to have had your wish than wish you had.

Taking Each Other for Granted

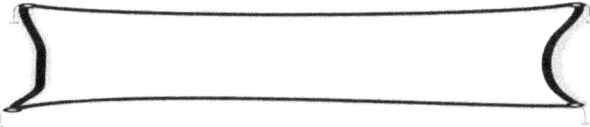

Each one of us has a goal in life – to be happy. I sincerely believe that you should get happiness out of small things in life or you will never know what happiness is. Giving due respect to each other and to your relationship will give you a deep sense of happiness whereas taking each other for granted will not only make life monotonous but it will also rob you of all the joys and pleasures of exploring new horizons.

Ranjan and Manju are married for six years now. Manju is a housewife and would sit the whole day in the house waiting for Ranjan to come back. Initially, Ranjan used to come back on time. Manju would then give all the details of her day's activities which Ranjan would listen amidst the sips of hot tea. But for sometime now, Ranjan has made it a habit to come home late, have dinner and go to sleep. Manju keeps waiting for him all evening. But he does not talk to her much. He takes Manju for granted. He knows she is there to cook, to look after his home and children. She feels as if he is treating her as a part of the furniture in the house which has been brought in and used to its maximum advantage. He does not talk to her or lend her a responsive ear either. Manju hates Ranjan's attitude but cannot help it. All that she can do is cry her heart out at night only to wake up to live another day with the same monotonous routine.

Look within yourself before you point a finger at your husband. He was not like this earlier. He gave you time and attention earlier but then you started taking him for granted. You would blabber off all your problems the moment he entered the house without even thinking that the poor tired soul might need some rest first. Grow up and learn to solve your own problems instead of telling your husband about the silly little difficulties of the day. Make it a rule not to tell your husband anything unpleasant till he has his tea and settled down. The heavens won't fall! If nothing happened the entire day, another half an hour will not make much of a difference. Your husband wants some peace of mind when he comes home.

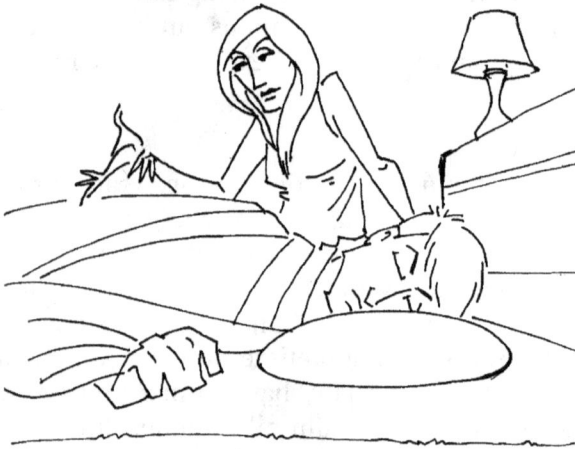

Do not nag, do not shout, do not pester. Do not take your relationship with your better half for granted. Do not throw tantrums. Let your husband relax after a day's hard work and enjoy those quiet moments together. Discuss your problems with him when he is in a better frame of mind. Give new dimensions to your relationship and it will fill your life with new happiness.

Think of all the good times both of you have spent together. Try to rekindle the same magic. Use soft music, soft lighting and good food to enhance his mood. Believe me, by the time, he is ready to listen to your problems, you too would be so relaxed that you will fi nd it inappropriate to mention them at this magic hour.

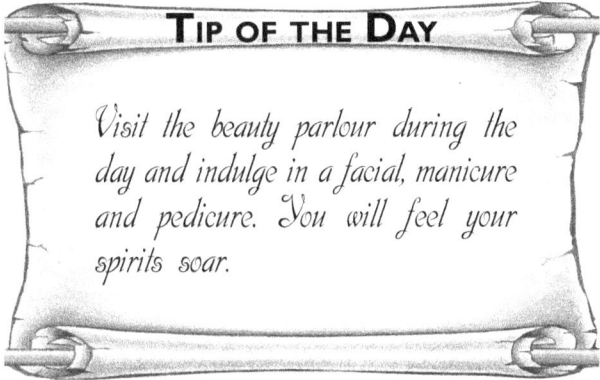

TIP OF THE DAY

Visit the beauty parlour during the day and indulge in a facial, manicure and pedicure. You will feel your spirits soar.

At Your Mercy

BUSTER 20

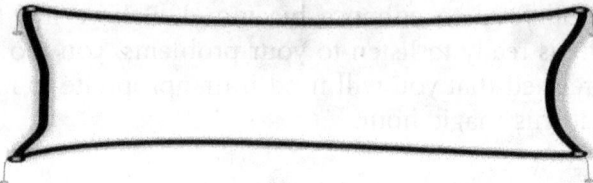

Dependence on your husband can certainly bring your stress levels to soar. You cannot control the other person. If you depend on him to a great extent then there are chances that he may not come up to your expectations each time. And every time, you fi nd a job unsatisfactory, you will get tensed because fi rst of all the work is pending and secondly, you feel cheated as your expectations were high due to your dependence on him for all matters.

Ranjita would depend upon her husband for fi xing things in the house, for taking her shopping, to deposit bills and many other sundry jobs. She would give the excuse that she did not know how to drive, so how could she move around? One day, when her husband was on tour, the kitchen faucet started leaking. She tried to put some cloth on it to stop the fl ow but nothing seemed to work. The more she tried, the worse it became. She called the plumber but he was out on call. The fl ow of water was so much that it had started seeping into the dining room threatening the precious rug. Ranjita was in a fi x when suddenly, the door bell rang. It was her neighbour, Sudha. Seeing her worried expression, Sudha enquired about the problem. When Ranjita told her, Sudha asked her to show the tap which was leaking. On seeing the tap, Sudha simply bent down and turned off the main supply to the faucet. In no time, the fl ow of water stopped and Ranjita heaved a sigh of relief. The two friends had a hearty laugh, but in her heart, Ranjita felt embarrassed for being so ignorant. If only she had taken some interest in things which she always thought to be a male-dominated territory then she would not have faced such a problem.

All the housewives are well educated today. So why depend upon your husband for doing menial work. With a little effort on your part you can very well handle jobs such as getting small things fi xed around the house, deposit electricity and telephone bills and do the weekly shopping for groceries. If you have a car, learn to drive. This will make you mobile and you will fell independent. Being on your own will help you complete the jobs on time and save you a lot of unnecessary tension.

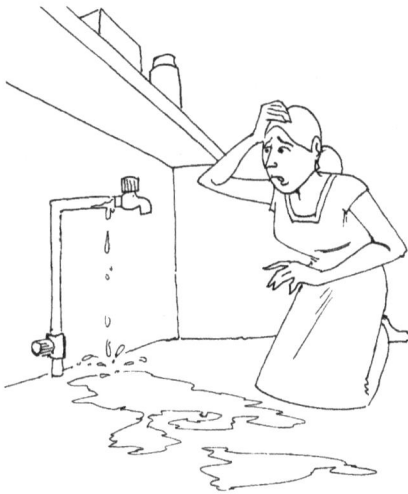

Why should you be at someone's mercy? Women are no less than men. There is no more division of territories now. If men can be the best cooks, why can't you be a plumber or an electrician for a change?

It is better to be independent so that you can organise your jobs according to their priorities and do them on time. Independence will bring new happiness in your life. You will feel more confi dent and self assured. And your hubby will admire you and welcome your new found status.

TIP OF THE DAY

There is bound to be a good way to get you in a good mood - you just have to find it.

Fix a mega sandwich.

Take a bath with essential oils.

Take a brisk walk.

Call a friend for a chat or

Repair something in the house.

You are My Confidante

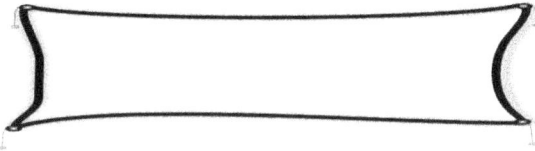

You could do well to remember that with your hubby, as in all human relationships, too much honesty can create problems. All delicately balanced relationships require us to blunt the sharp cutting edge of truth with diplomacy and tact.

When Shuchi was in college, she fell in love with a muslim boy. Since her parents were totally against the match, she sacrificed her love and agreed to marry the boy of her parent's choice. Anil was a handsome young man who was very loving. Shuchi was besotted by his charms. They got along well too. They got married amidst much fanfare and soon after, they headed to Shimla for their honeymoon.

During some intimate and emotional moments, Shuchi admitted to Anil, about her affair with a muslim boy. While coaxing her in telling him all her love affairs before marriage, Anil had promised not to take it to heart.

But once the truth was out, he could not digest the fact that his wife was in love with someone else before marriage. Their ten-day long honeymoon was shrunk to two days and they were back home, the third day itself.

Shuchi began her married life on shaky grounds just because she forgot to blunt the sharp edge of truth.

Your husband may be your best friend, still there are a few things which are best unsaid. Put yourself in your husband's place and imagine your own reaction to such outbursts. Since our childhood, we have been taught to be honest and never to tell a lie. But a lie is not a lie if it is told for something good. So understand the temperament and psychology of your husband and act accordingly. Do not just blabber whatever comes to your mind. Be tactful and let peace prevail.

In your life, you will be faced with many such situations where you will have to think twice before uttering the truth. In such cases, it is better to be tactful than to spoil your relations by telling the truth. Your husband may be very caring, understanding and a true angel still there may be a weak spot in his heart, which you may hurt by being blunt about a touching subject.

Ignorance is bliss. What you do not know does not hurt you.

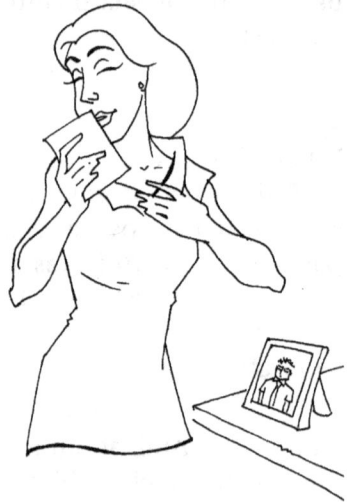

TIP OF THE DAY

Open the windows. Let the light shine through and the energy flow freely.

Pati Parmeshwar

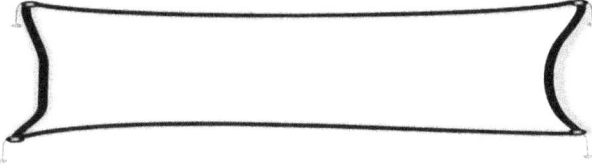

God made men and women equal. Over the years, our system adopted the fact that man is superior to woman, primarily because a man is physically stronger than a woman. But when you marry, you marry for love. And two people are always at par in love.

Sugandha was a well educated girl with modern views. She got married in a rich but orthodox family. Her in-laws lived in Bikaner. They had a family business which was jointly run by her father-in-law and her husband who was their only son. Everything was fine till that fateful day when Sugandha discovered that her husband was addicted to vices like drinking, gambling and also visited brothels. She was shocked and raised a hue and cry in the house.

She thought, her husband who was so affectionate till now will understand and promise to amend his ways. But her mother-in-law came to her son's rescue and started preaching Sugandha on the significance of *Pati Parmeshwar*.

First, she tried to pacify Sugandha, when she refused to give in, she got angry and told Sugandha to shut up in clear terms. She said, "Your *Pati* is your God. How dare you raise your voice against him?" Sugandha was stunned. If she were wrong, would her husband have forgiven her so easily?

Your husband is a human being just like you. Why accord him the status of God if he does not deserve it? You are two individuals married to each other with a number of vices and virtues. Why not accept each other as human beings and try to amend the faults in each other? However, turning a blind eye to all your husband's faults just because he is your *Pati Parmeshwar* is not correct.

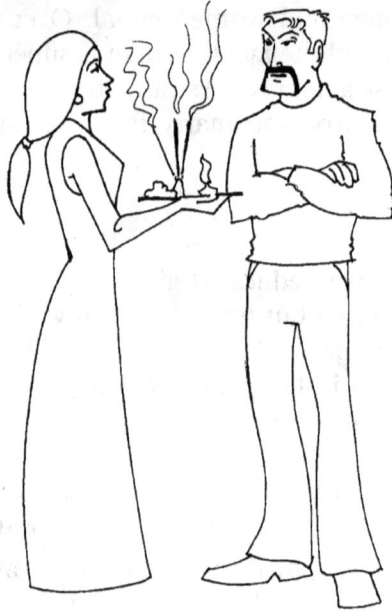

Gone are the days when a husband was considered to be God by his wife. Today, both are on equal footing. So giving the status of God to the husband is neither advisable nor practical. He is as much a human being as you are, so why give this special treatment to him and create unnecessary stress in the house?

Your husband is your partner for life. He comes from the same mould in which you are made. Love him, adore him, fi ght with him, care for him, but do not worship him. That puts him on a pedestal so high up that you may not be able to relate to him normally.

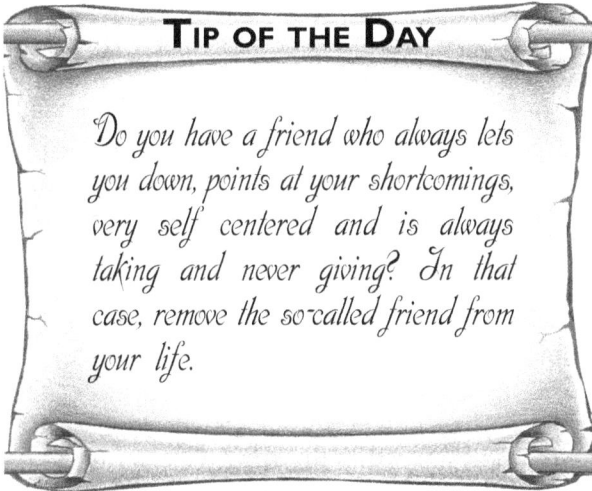

TIP OF THE DAY

Do you have a friend who always lets you down, points at your shortcomings, very self centered and is always taking and never giving? In that case, remove the so-called friend from your life.

Extramarital Affairs

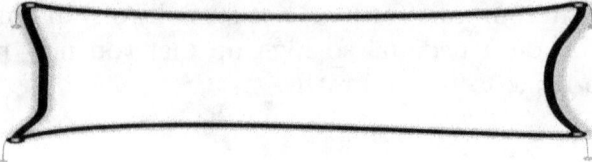

Marriage is a commitment for life. Infidelity in marriage is not acceptable. There are many causes for indulging into extramarital affairs. There may be conflicts between the spouses. There may be heated exchanges which turn hostile. Then there may be a communication gap. Silence, at times, harbours internal seething which may erupt anytime. Then there are sexual adjustments which form the very basis of a marriage. Maladjustments in this area pose marital risk. Spouses may turn rebellious giving way to extra marital relationships. The biggest problem is the personal attitude of one or both the partners. People fail to understand their own feelings. They fail to appreciate the love in their lives. They fail to understand that marriage is a lifelong relationship where the couple should be committed to each other.

Rishita's husband was having an affair with his secretary. When Rishita came to know about it, she was aghast. She could not believe her ears. But when she saw the two of them coming out of a hotel room like a lovey-dovey couple, there was no room left for doubt. Her world was shattered. She had two small children to look after and she was not earning either. She was totally dependent on her husband for everything. What would she do? If she encounters him, he may decide to leave her for that woman. And if she kept quite, her conscience pricked her. The stress was killing her.

In such a situation, children are your biggest assets. Every father loves his children and feels responsible towards them. He would defi nitely not want to deprive them of his love and affection. Do not involve the children in the matter, but rest assured that half your battle is won. Now look at the other things. Delve on the areas which could have led him to go astray. Is it your behaviour towards him, is your appearance not very appealing, have you put on too much weight, have you lost him because you could not keep the magic alive in your marriage? etc. Find out the reason behind his going to the other woman, and try to rectify it.

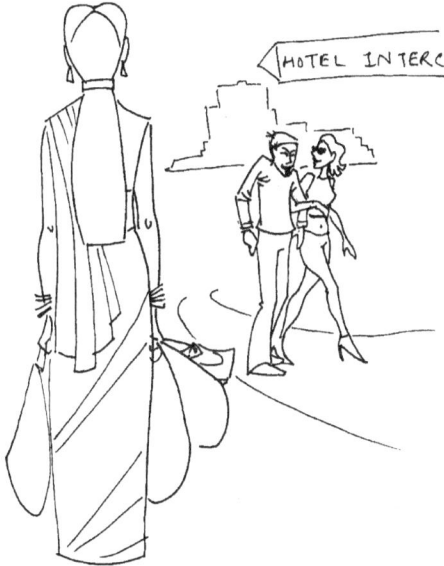

Extramarital affairs can certainly take their toll on you. It is like a jolt to your ego. It shakes you up completely. The person whom you always thought belonged to you, is now shared by someone else too. This stress is enough to take you into the deep valleys of depression. But crying or feeling stressed is not the solution to this problem. Look for the areas in which you lack, and which could have led your man to go astray. If you rectify your faults then there are less chances of your man going away from you.

Consider a situation, in which a husband comes home from a day's hard work. He feels like relaxing over a cup of tea with a refreshing chat with his wife. But what he gets in return is a frown on her face, a list of complaints and a much delayed tea. Instead of sharing the day's events, his wife gives a long list of troubles created by the children during the day. The fi nal straw comes when she hands him over the shopping list. To escape her fury, the poor man goes to the market much against his wishes to buy the grocery. All this is unnecessary stress which could have been avoided. Such situations may lead to the man staying away from home for longer hours and may end up with an extramarital affair.

It's never too late to try. He has loved you, and he still loves you. It's only lust that has taken over for the time being. He will defi nitely come back to you with some efforts on your part.

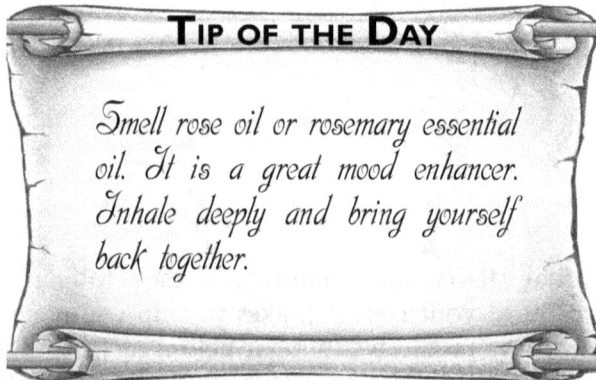

TIP OF THE DAY

Smell rose oil or rosemary essential oil. It is a great mood enhancer. Inhale deeply and bring yourself back together.

Stress in Social Life

One day Akbar was simply chatting with his friends, who were the best, wisest, most creative people chosen from every part of the country. They were amidst serious discussion when Akbar slapped Birbal – for no apparent reason. Now one could not slap the Emperor back, but the slap had to go somewhere. So Birbal slapped the person who was sitting next to him. They were all wise people still they could not comprehend the reason for the slaps going around. Because Akbar slapped Birbal out of the blue and Birbal instead of enquiring from the Emperor as to why he slapped him, slapped the man by his side.

Now that man, thinking perhaps this was the norm at the court, slapped the next person. In a chain reaction, the slap went around the court.

That night, the queen slapped Emperor Akbar in their bedroom. Stunned, Akbar asked, "Why did you slap me?"

The queen said, "What a question – a game is a game."

Akbar asked, "Who told you that this is a game?" The queen replied, "We have been hearing the whole day long that a great game has begun in the court. The only rule is you cannot hit the person back. You have to find somebody else to slap. Now somebody has slapped me – so your slap has come back to you. The game is now complete."

Akbar did not know what to say, so he kept mum.

Everything comes back to its source.

You spread goodness, it brings you reward.

You spread evil, you get punishment in return.

This is the fundamental rule of life,

The world is a stage where we all are actors playing our designated roles. What is important is that how well we play our roles and not the role itself.

Friends Forever

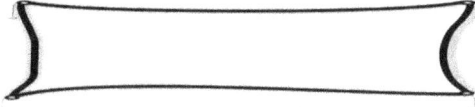

Friends are our biggest assets. To have a good friend is like having something precious which will last a lifetime. It is said, that we cannot choose our parents, our relatives, our siblings, but friends – we can choose them. So naturally, they are closer to our heart. A woman's best friend is her husband. But there are certain things which she cannot confi de even in him. This is where a friend steps in.

Shruti and Shyama were good friends. They would confi de in each other. There would be endless conversations on phone once their husbands went to work. By quirk of fate, it so happened that Shruti's husband started seeing another woman. By the time, Shruti came to know about it, he was already much deep into the affair. Shruti would cry her heart out to Shyama. Shyama felt sorry for her friend. Her husband, Ritesh also sympathized with Shruti. Soon it became a routine. Shruti would cry her woes to Shyama during the day which Shyama passed on to Ritesh in the evening when he came back from work. Shyama would only talk about Shruti and her problems. Soon Ritesh was sick of all this.

One day, when he could not stand it any longer, he told Shyama to either put an end to it or he may take the clue and fi nd solace outside home. Shyama was shocked at Ritesh's outburst. She had not bargained for this stress which she was unknowingly building in her family life.

As a true friend, if you listen to your friend's woes and try to help her out then you are really a kind person. But if your own life is getting affected due to this, then it is time to take a quick look. If all your conversations with your husband end up with your friend's tales of woes then it may bring stress in your own relationship. After coming back from office, the tired husband would want to share his day with you rather than listening to your friend's silly fights with her husband or mother-in-law. So keep your friends and their problems to yourself and do not spoil your own love life because of this.

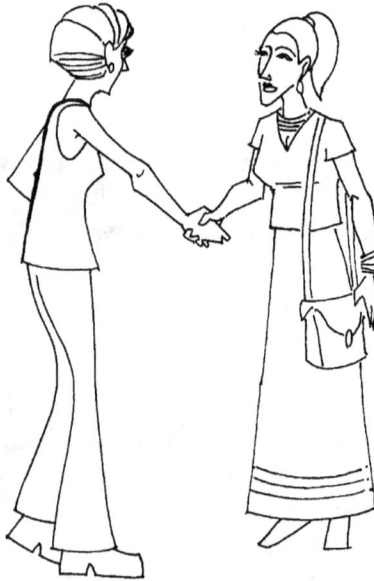

Nothing is really lost. All you need is a little restrain on your emotions and check on your tongue. Discuss your friends with your husband but not always the ones who are facing problems. After putting in a hard day at office, your husband deserves some freshness and some light hearted chatter from you.

Poor guy, your husband that is, has been working hard. So don't break him, just give him a break.

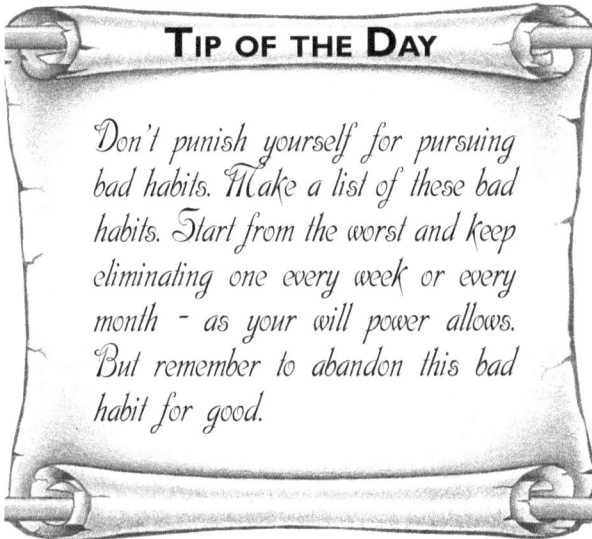

TIP OF THE DAY

Don't punish yourself for pursuing bad habits. Make a list of these bad habits. Start from the worst and keep eliminating one every week or every month – as your will power allows. But remember to abandon this bad habit for good.

Stepping Beyond Limits

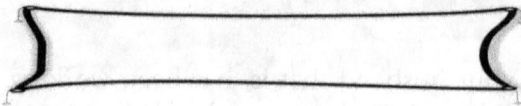

Neighbours, friends and kitty parties form an integral part of our daily life for most housewives. It is a virtue, they should not be denied as they too need some moments of recreation. But what should be avoided is excessive indulgence in them.

When Rachit shifted to a posh area of the city, he had not bargained for the mounting expenses by way of kitty parties which his wife Supriya indulged. He was a man of modest means. His company provided him this house, but his earnings remained the same. All the other ladies in Supriya's kitty party were from rich families. They could easily afford the kitty of five thousand rupees per month. But for Supriya, who belonged to the middle class, it was a big amount. To be in the group, Supriya joined the kitty beyond her means. She started dishing out this huge sum every month. It proved too much for her budget. By her sixth kitty, Supriya had already exhausted all her savings. For her next kitty, Supriya had just a thousand rupees left from household expenses. She took out four thousand rupees kept by Rachit for Diwali expenses and went to the party. Later when Ruchit opened the cupboard to take out the money to buy crackers and other goodies for Diwali, he was shocked to find the money missing. A sheepish Supriya admitted taking the money for her kitty. She told him to withdraw money from his fixed deposit in the Bank. Rachit was very angry to hear this. He refused to delve into his hard earned savings. That year they did not celebrate Diwali at all. A tense atmosphere hung in the house.

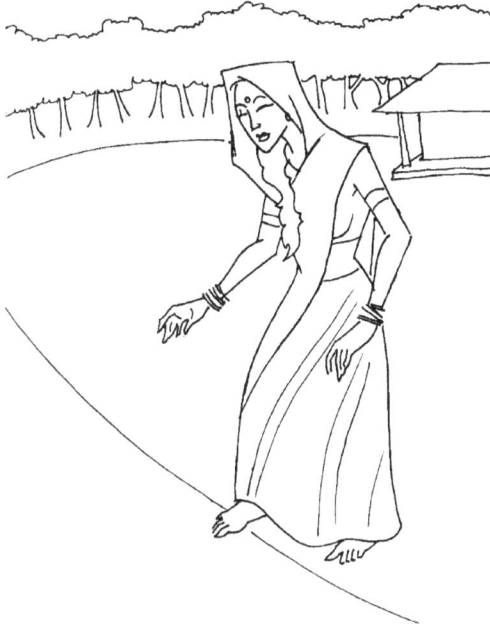

If you are a member of such kitty parties which are beyond your means then that will create tension in the house. You may find it difficult to squeeze a high amount for the kitty every month. Apart from that, you also have to take care of other things like new clothes, trendy accessories and lunch or dinner expenses too. All this can burn a big hole in your pocket if you do not belong to the some bracket as that other kitty members do. So if you are so keen on joining a kitty party, then it is better to join the one which is within your limits. Getting into something which does not suit you, just for the heck of it is not a wise idea. This can even give rise to unnecessary scuffles with your spouse too.

Keep away from such stressors which are unnecessary in life. Try spending your time in doing other constructive activities. If you want to interact with people, you may join an NGO or a welfare organization which would not only give you a better exposure, but also give you the satisfaction of doing a good deed.

Know your priorities. Do not go beyond your means and create tension for everyone.

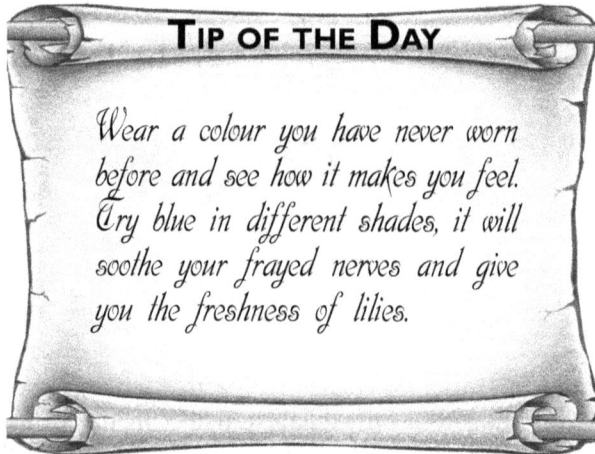

TIP OF THE DAY

Wear a colour you have never worn before and see how it makes you feel. Try blue in different shades, it will soothe your frayed nerves and give you the freshness of lilies.

Showing off Wealth

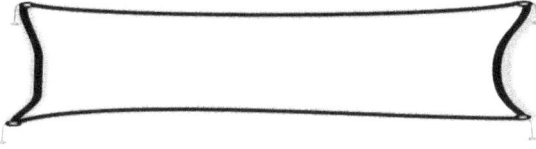

What a lovely diamond ring, when did you buy it?

"I have just come back from a month long Europe tour."

"Look at Mrs. Chaddha, what a snob she is."

The above ....are some common snippets from a kitty party or any gathering of women. Showing off their wealth is a common phenomenon among housewives who meet once or twice a month. If you are not from an affl uent family, but you have joined such groups then these get togethers are likely to make you tense as you will feel out of place and not up to it.

Some moments ago, we read about Supriya and Rachit. Supriya was stuck in the vicious circle of expensive Kitty parties, money and the means. On the face of it, you may feel that Supriya was greatly enjoying these parties. Come let's take a look at one such party and you will realise how unfi t Supriya felt in these parties, yet she kept attending them to maintain her social status and to be able to boast about her connection with the group of ladies.

All the women who were the members of that kitty party would arrive in their shining new cars even if they lived at a walking distance from the host member's house. Supriya would generally take a lift from a member who lived in her neighbourhood on the pretext that her husband had an important meeting to attend so he took the car. Each party saw the women in new sarees, latest outfits and a different set of jewellery. Supriya wore her best saree twice with a gap of three kitties thinking that no one would notice. But the women there were smarter than she thought. They would pinpoint immediately.

Their talks always revolved around five star hotels, holiday resorts and foreign trips. Supriya never indulged in any such luxuries so either she kept a pretense or avoided the topic. All in all, Supriya felt a total misfit for these parties but since she wanted to be with the in-group, she dared not leave the kitty.

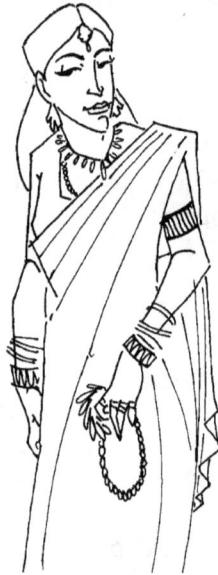

However, the truth remaineds that each time she had to go for a kitty party, she would be more tense than happy — the tension of arranging for the kitty money, new clothes and matching jewellery, transport, trips to the beauty parlour — all this would leave her exhausted.

One way out is to avoid such groups and join other people who are more of your kind. Another way is you keep the pretense and fl ow with the tide. "Who is going to check"? – Keep this phrase in mind and let go of your imagination. The fi rst way is secure and is sure to restore your peace of mind whereas in the other way, you will have to bear the burden of uttering a pack of lies. This will increase your levels of anxiety.

As I said before, this is an unnecessary stress. In the end, you are not going to gain anything. You are so impressed with these rich women, but if you ask them what are their achievements, they would not be able to answer. What they have been doing all their lives is spending their husband's hard earned money for their worldly pleasures. Their home and kids are looked after by servants. They are not even fulfi lling their duty as wife, what would they talk of achievements?

In his wisdom, God gives to each of us a limited number of hours in which to achieve our goals. Whatever success we may achieve in this life will come from the purpose to which we put God's priceless gift – time.

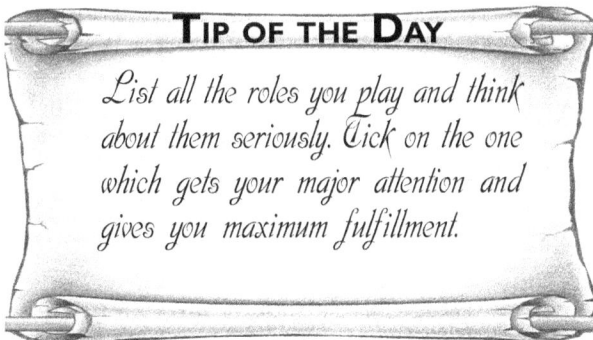

TIP OF THE DAY

List all the roles you play and think about them seriously. Tick on the one which gets your major attention and gives you maximum fulfillment.

Neglecting Home

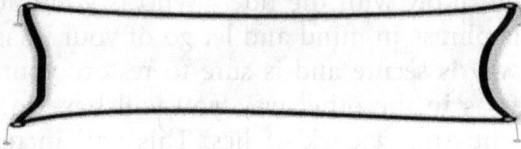

If you are neglecting home to go to these kitty parties or indulge in gossip sessions, then there are bound to have problems at home. Your husband, children and your in- laws, who feel neglected will certainly complain giving rise to tensions in the family.

Ridhima was a fun loving girl. Even after she became the mother of two children, her friend circle did not shrink. Since her in-laws lived with her, she passed on the responsibility of her children to them while she went out with her friends to enjoy her innumerous cards sessions or shopping sprees. She hired a cook so that she was not tied with cooking. She clearly neglected her home but no one would dare say anything to her as she had a bad temper. Once it so happened that her sister-in-law, who lived in a nearby town, fell ill so both her mother-in-law and father-in-law went to see her. That day Ridhima went to her card party as usual. She left the cook at home and instructed her to lock the house before she left. The children were to return from school by three o' clock. Her card session went on till half past three. Obviously, she missed their school bus. When she remembered, she rushed home only to fi nd the kids sobbing outside the locked house. Realizing that the cook must have left, she consoled the children and opened the lock with her own key. What lay before her eyes was a sight worst than her sobbing kids. The whole house was ransacked and all the valuables were missing. The cook had vanished with all her precious things. Ridhima had to pay dearly for her careless attitude. Her in-laws and her husband rebuked her and for once, Ridhima had no words but only tears in her eyes.

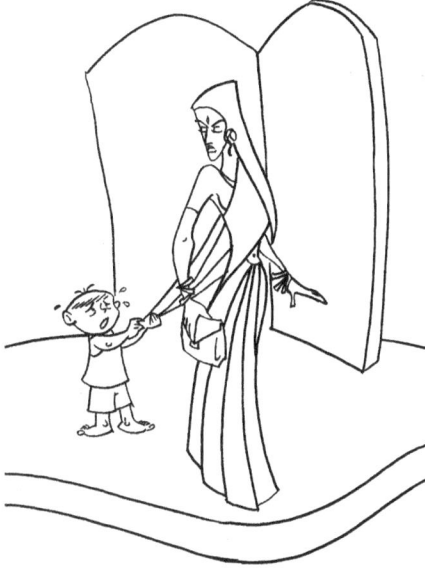

To overcome this problem, the simple solution lies in your own hands. Stop neglecting your duties at home. Give ample time to your family and kids. A perfect balance between your home and recreation is what is needed to keep all stress at bay.

Neglecting children and husband for playing cards or for shopping or indulging in gossip for long hours will not take you anywhere. Ultimately, its your own life which will suffer. Remember, your home is your *Karambhoomi*. If you do not perform your *karma* religiously, then you ought to suffer. But if you are not neglecting your duties, then it is your right to get that bit of enjoyment to which you are truly entitled.

It is not being selfish to aim for your happiness with some amount of common sense. So make your family happy first, yourself next. You will find your happiness being doubled in this way.

TIP OF THE DAY

If you want happiness for an hour, take a nap.

If you want happiness for a day, go on a picnic.

If you want happiness for a week, go on a vacation.

If you want happiness for a month, be a spendthrift.

If you want happiness for a year, construct a house.

If you want happiness for a lifetime, nurture your family with love and care.

Bitchy Neighbours

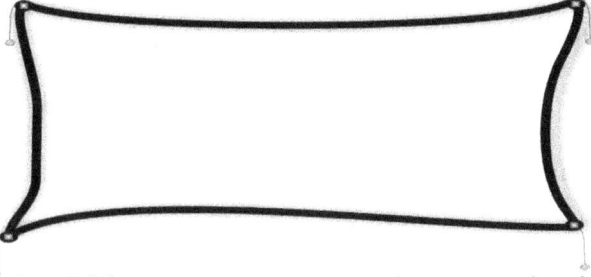

Good neighbours act as are our insurance in time of adversity. People who live in a good neighbourhood would vouch for it. If we are blessed with good neighbours, we should consider ourselves lucky.

Neighbours not only share your joys, they also console you in your time of sorrow. They lend colour to a celebration by joining in your merry making. They also support you in a mishap. However, as all fingers in a hand are not equal, similarly, not all neighbours are good. You may come across bitchy neighbours as well who would cause stress in your life.

Saroj and her neighbours always enjoyed their tete-a-tete after finishing their morning chores. They would assemble at the central park of the colony and share each other's thoughts and problems. It was a good company till Santo mausi moved in the colony. Santo Mausi was Saroj's widowed aunt. She had no children so she decided to move in with her niece. Santo Mausi was a great gossip monger and trouble shooter. She would poke her nose into everyone's affair. After each morning session in the park, she could be seen visiting some household or the other on the pretext of having a friendly chat. There she would bitch about other neighbours swearing to tell only the truth. These things led to fights and episodes of verbal encounters among the otherwise friendly neighbours. The unpleasantness among the neighbours soon became evident, and the congenial assembly in the park was abandoned since almost everyone was at loggerheads with the other. The tension between the neighbours heightened with time and soon the men and children were dragged into it. The lively central park now bore a deserted look. Saroj and her friends missed those golden days which were now just a thing of past.

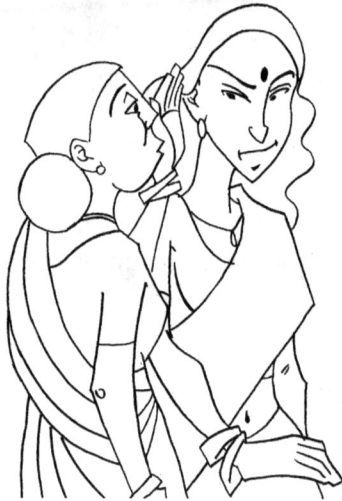

It is a common practice among housewives to meet after finishing the morning chores for a chit chat. It is good so long as the talks are restricted to general topics and not about anyone in particular. It is also a good means of recreation and to curb boredom. But if you start bitching about people or enjoy the gossip, then such sessions may give you stress. It also leaves you open to speculation and mars your reputation in the eyes of people.

Using your own discretion while dealing with people shall help you assess the other person's intentions. If you are ever in doubt about the truth, it's better to check it out yourself rather than believing in others. Never ever utter wrong words for anyone because you never know how your words may be twisted and taken to the other party.

Neighbours are your assets, but do not let them turn into your liabilities. Maintain congenial relations with them, but keep a distance.

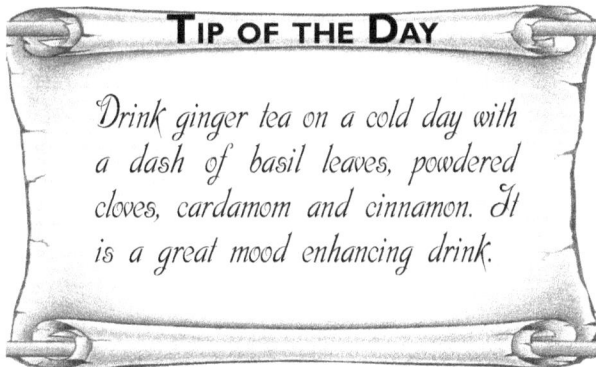

TIP OF THE DAY

Drink ginger tea on a cold day with a dash of basil leaves, powdered cloves, cardamom and cinnamon. It is a great mood enhancing drink.

Transfer Blues

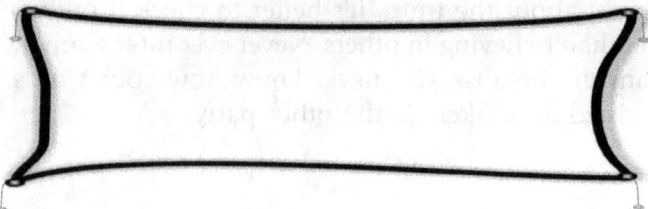

Even though you are not working, your life can be full of stressors if your husband has a transferable job. Travelling can be fun for some, but it can be tiresome for others.

If your husband is in a transferable job, there are many factors which can act as stressors. First of all, not been able to settle down properly in one place. Then the tension of packing and unpacking every now and then. If children are there, then their education also suffers because of transfers. The damage to the furniture and other things during transfers can also cause considerable stress to a housewife who has built her home with love and care.

Shalini was married to an army offi cer. When she got married, her husband was posted on a non-family station. After a few months, he got his posting at a family station and was allotted a family residential quarter, she moved in enthusiastically. In her enthusiasm, she bought the best furniture and other household goods. But her enthusiasm evaporated when she realized that it was tough packing and unpacking things every few years.

With children arriving, she was hardly left with any energy to carry her precious luggage with her. She got so disgusted with moving every now and then that she started dreading the transfer orders.

In Shalini's case, initially, her husband watched her as a mute spectator. Then one day, he advised her to dispose off all the heavy furniture and buy some light cane furniture. Reluctantly, she agreed. But this eased her burden so much that each time, she started selling her earlier furniture before the posting and buying new cheaper stuff at the next station.

She found this more invigorating and refreshing. Today, she loves moving on and looks forward to her husband's transfer orders.

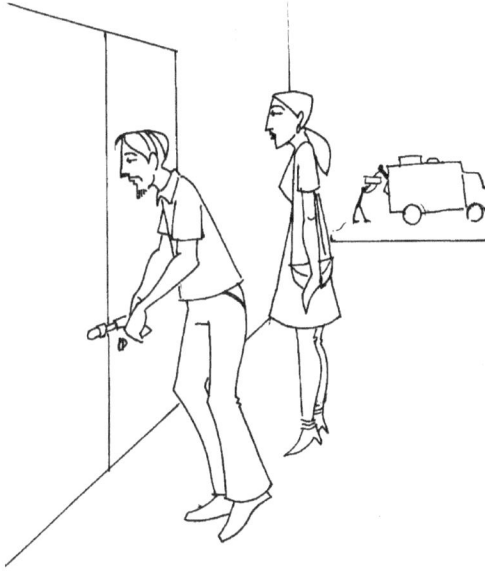

Getting stressed over packing or fussing over other trivial matters will only create tension in the house. So look at the positive side of the things. Take it as an opportunity to break the monotony of daily life. Think in positive terms and enjoy the prospective of redecorating your house.

Life moves on, so do we. So why get stressed over something which is a part of our lives? Keeping your mind free from all the tension while travelling or while shifting residence will make your experience novel and more enjoyable.

TIP OF THE DAY

Want to lose weight instantly! Check your key ring. Do you use all the keys still? Get rid of all the keys from the previous house and the ones you do not use anymore. You don't need to carry the excess weight around each day. Happy weight loss.

Bringing up Children

*A*kbar once saw a woman hugging and kissing a child that did not look particularly appealing. Akbar expressed surprise that a woman could lavish so much love on such an unattractive child.

"That's because it's her own child", explained Birbal, "to a mother her child is the most beautiful in the world."

"How can that be", the emperor was not satisfied by Birbal's explanation.

The next day, Birbal called a guard and in the presence of Emperor Akbar ordered him to bring the most beautiful child to the palace.

The following day, the guard came to the palace with a small boy with buck teeth and hair that stood up like porcupine quills and hesitantly pushed him in front of Akbar.

"The most beautiful child, Your Majesty." He said in a hesitant voice.

"How do you know he is beautiful?" asked Akbar.

"My wife, his mother, says so." Replied the guard.

There is no arguing with a mother's love. It is consistent and unshakeable. Nothing can suppress it. If we can be half as consistent in our relationships and in our dealings with our dear ones, half our problems will be solved.

Kiddies Corner

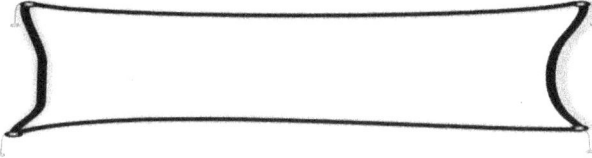

*C*hildren spell responsibility and no responsibility is free of stress and worry. Bringing up children is a matter of joy with some traces of stress and worries.

This is perhaps the best phase in a housewife's life. In many cases, motherhood is the deciding factor for a woman choosing to be a housewife. This is the beginning of a new life for the mother and the child, both. When the baby is small, the mother keeps worrying about his growth, eating pattern, etc. She spends sleepless nights to meet the demands of the infant. Cooperation from the family members boosts her morale and she does not feel fatigued or stressed. But if she does not get any support from her husband or in-laws, then the situation becomes very tiring for her. The joy of motherhood turns into stressful moments of despair.

Nita got married to the younger son of the Malhotra household. Her elder sister-in-law had a two-year old son. A year later, Nita also gave birth to a baby boy. Celebrations fi lled the house with joy and laughter. Everyone was happy. As time passed, Nita's son started growing and started crossing each milestone of childhood. Nita felt happy to see her baby growing. But there was a problem, each time her baby would miss a milestone even by a month, her mother-in-law would start comparing him with the elder sister-in-law's son. "Aditya started smiling when he was just two weeks old, why hasn't Abhishek started smiling till now?

He is almost a month old now", or Aditya cut his first tooth in the fifth month, but Abhishek is in his seventh month now, still no signs of cutting teeth, etc." The comparison irked Nita very much. Although, each time she consulted the pediatrician about Abhishek's progress, he would give a satisfying nod. Still a doubt lurched in her mind because of the comparisons made by her mother-in-law. She felt as if her son was a laggard and it made her restless and tense.

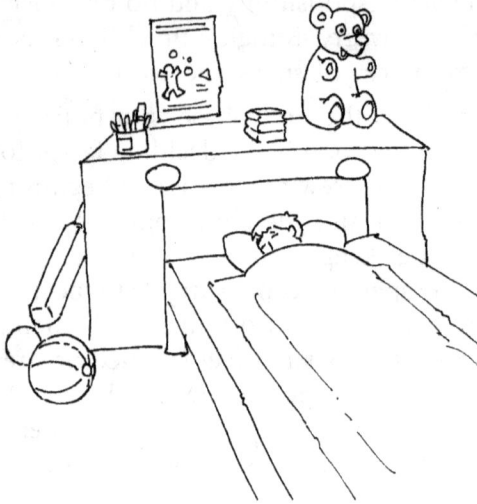

"My child started walking when she was nine months old" or "she spoke her first words before she cut her first tooth" and so on. The list is endless. Every mother takes pride in her children's achievements. There are milestones set by doctors for the baby's growth taking an average child in consideration. So if your child did not manage to achieve some of these milestones, don't fret. Getting agitated over such trivial matters will be of no use. Remember, all children are not alike. Some are fast learners, while some are slow learners. But sooner or later, they all come round and grow up into normal, healthy children.

The role of parents is a unique one. Do not compare your children's growth with others. And if others do so then do not feel bad about it. You cannot stop anyone from voicing their opinion. Have faith in your child, God and your genes. You will sail through.

After you are through with this phase and you look back in retrospect, then you will fi nd yourself smiling at your own foolishness. The stress which you experienced at that time was of no consequence – this you will realise later.

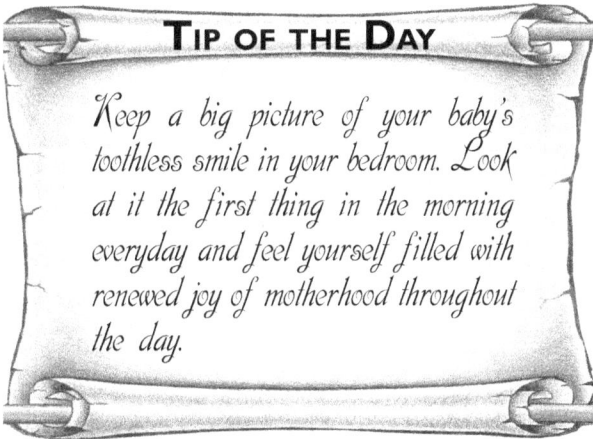

TIP OF THE DAY

Keep a big picture of your baby's toothless smile in your bedroom. Look at it the first thing in the morning everyday and feel yourself filled with renewed joy of motherhood throughout the day.

High Expectations

Small children depend on their mothers for each and every thing. It is a delight for them to have their mother around them. That is why a homemaker plays a very important role in shaping the future of her children. But remember one thing, never expect anything from anybody. This includes your children too. Children are like delicate, innocent buds which are yet to bloom. Expecting them to show results before time is asking too much from them.

Ria was Sudha's only child. She was quite intelligent. Sudha had high expectations from her. When Ria was young, Sudha enrolled her in various hobby classes so that she could become an all rounder. Ria would go for swimming, painting, dance and music classes regularly besides attending normal school. During summer vacation, her routine would be very tight, what with more hobby courses like computer, creative writing, western dance and music, clay modelling, etc., keeping the little girl busy throughout the day. Ria would have loved to play 'ghar-ghar' with her friends, but Sudha forced her to play games like—chess, monopoly and scrabble. During Ria's Xth board exams, Sudha was continuously hovering around her coaxing her to study. The results were far from satisfying. Sudha was devastated. As she was about to reprimand her daughter on such low grades, she was met with a gory sight on entering Ria's bedroom. Ria had committed suicide by hanging herself to the ceiling.

Sudha's world came crashing down. What had she gained by putting so much pressure on her poor child all these years? A good life was wasted due to the stress and tensions which were pressed on to the child through the mother.

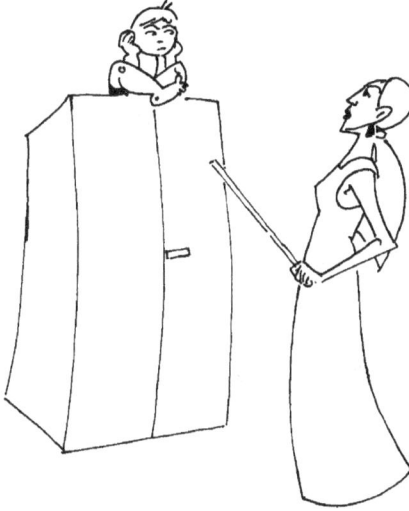

Never keep your expectations too high. Treat your child as an average child. Reward them with your biggest hug if they achieve something, but do not punish them for not achieving something. We see many cases around us where either parents or children themselves went into depression for not having achieved the desired targets. Please don't play in the hands of fate. Keep your cool and let life take its own course. Remember, 'all's well that ends well.'

Children are your assets, don't turn them into your liabilities. Give them time and space to spread their wings. Life of a housewife is full of stress. Starting from the birth of her child to the day the child grows up into an adult, the housewife experiences stress in different forms. But living with stress for such a long time is not good. So it's better for her to manage her stress levels by taking a positive and relaxed view of life instead of passing it on to her children.

They are your children not slaves. You brought them into this world but you did not give them life. So why try to control it?

TIP OF THE DAY

Keeping energy levels high is very important.

Eat your first meal within an hour of the day to keep your energy levels optimum. Your last meal should be taken four hours before bedtime so that the body has enough time to digest the food.

Am I a Servant?

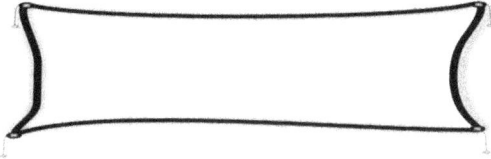

The love, care and protection that a housewife provides in the growing years of her children can never be substituted by a maid, grandparents or a creche as in the case of a working woman. But once children grow up, they start weaving their own world. They get too engrossed within their own group of friends, studies and outings. Unwittingly, they start distancing themselves from the mother. As they grow, they start detesting the caring attitude of their mother and take it as an interference in their independent way of living. In such a case, the poor mother, who has spent many years tending her kids feels at a loss and does not know where she went wrong. All of a sudden, stress crops within her. She feels hurt and dejected but does not find an escape route for her emotions.

Sunita was a village girl. She married Satish who was an electrician in Patna. In a few years, she became the mother of a son and a daughter. In the meantime, Satish got a good job in Mumbai and the family shifted there. They lived in a chawl. It was a new experience for Sunita. Satish admitted the children in good schools. Time passed by. Satish's work expanded and the family shifted to their own small house in the suburbs. The children were in college now. They spoke fluent English and wore trendy clothes. But there was a major change in their behaviour. They would treat their mother very badly. Sunita could neither speak nor understand English.

Her children started treating her as a servant. They would shout at her slightest mistake and make fun of her in English which she could not understand. Although Satish was also not very educated, still the children feared him because he was the provider of the family. Sunita would cry her heart out when alone, but she loved her children dearly so she never said anything to them. But the tension of being treated badly was taking its toll on her health.

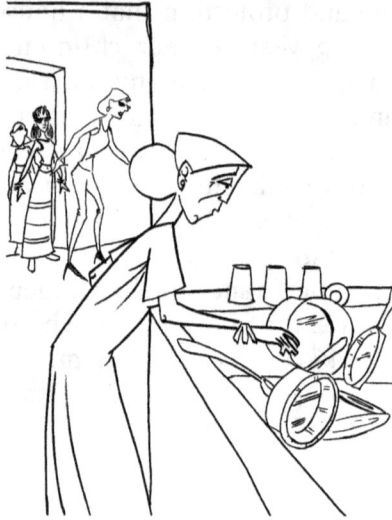

The worst part of her dilemma arrived when she was needed only for the housework in the house. Apart from that, her adolescent children treated her badly. In her mind, this kind of behaviour automatically transformed her from a housewife and a mother to a mere servant.

And the worst part was that she couldn't share this pain and feeling of hurt with anyone because it had been infl icted upon her by her own loved ones.

Getting your husband into confidence is a good idea. Being the stronger of the two parents, he can easily make the children see sense and correct their wrong behaviour. Remember living with stress for a long time is not good. So it's better for you to manage your stress levels soon by taking a positive and relaxed view of life.

Be strong. They are your children. You have brought them up. Why should you take all this rubbish from them? Be a no nonsense mother and show them who is the boss around here.

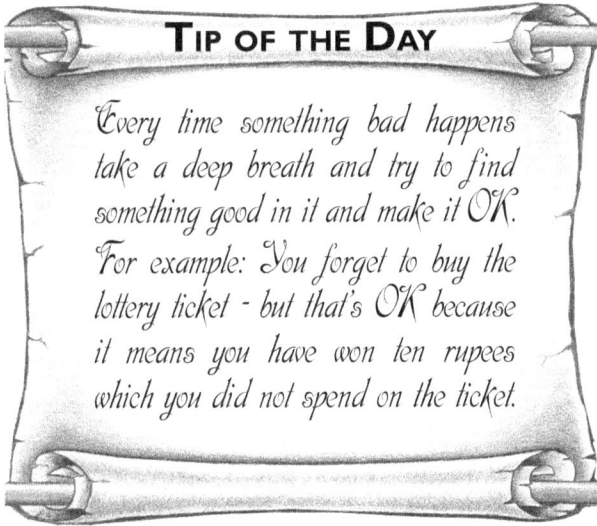

TIP OF THE DAY

Every time something bad happens take a deep breath and try to find something good in it and make it OK. For example: You forget to buy the lottery ticket - but that's OK because it means you have won ten rupees which you did not spend on the ticket.

Handling Adolescents

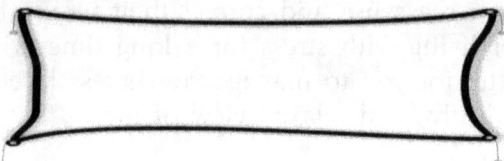

As children grow, it becomes diffi cult to handle them. As adolescents, they turn into a bunch of rebels who need to be tamed tactfully from time to time. Adolescence is a very crucial juncture for children. They should be handled properly otherwise they may turn astray.

My cousin, Rima has two teenaged daughters. They were very loving, affectionate and obedient till they were in school. Once I went to her house. Her daughters had joined college by then. As I sat enquiring about her daughters, one of them entered the room. Apparently, she was going to college. What surprised me most were her clothes and the manner in which she carried herself. She was wearing a skimpy top and skin tight trousers. She wished me by nodding and spoke to her mother in a very gruff voice. Gone was the plain, simple, homely sweet girl, I had seen the last time. She had come to borrow some money. In a jiffy, she was out of the house. Before I could ask anything from my cousin, she broke down. She told me how her daughter had changed since she joined college. While she was blaming the college and her friends for everything, I kept on thinking about the other girls who go to college and still retain their values and traditions. The girl was obviously not guided properly by the parents. It was later revealed by the mother, that she had been very strict with her daughters from the very beginning for the fear that they do not fall in bad company. She had put them in a girl's school, never allowed them to interact with boys and always kept their reins tightly in her hands. Till the daughters were in school, there was not much exposure, and they remained within limits. But college opened new horizons for them and now they felt free to fl y as they wished. They stopped bowing to the strict rules laid by their mother. 'What would happen to her daughters?' — This thought would nag Rima day and night and she felt miserable.

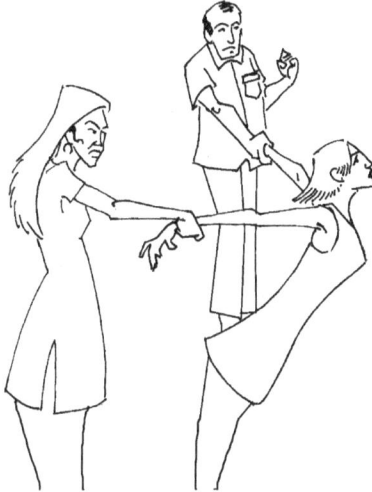

When you get stressed over your adolescent's behaviour, it is easier to blame squarely on the children. But we, as parents, too have a part to play. On our part, we should also allow youngsters some breathing space. Be an emotional anchor to them whenever they need it. Help them choose a satisfying career and stand by their decision. It is a rapidly changing world. You should give them little time to adapt, to make their choices, to follow their dreams. It's true that children are not always correct, nor are you. So learn to accept your mistakes in front of them. This will teach them modesty and they will also willingly admit their own mistakes. After making all these efforts, you are most likely to share a congenial relationship. Hence, the stress is managed automatically and in the most effi cient manner.

Once in a while, all children bring their friends home. So when adolescent children bring their friends home, why should you feel perturbed? College life is much diverse. Children from all over the country come and study together. Naturally, they have different styles, moves and philosophies. Feeling stressed over this matter will not be of any use. You should have confidence in your own child.

Children are your heart and soul. They should be nurtured with love and care. Instead of eyeing all their actions suspiciously, have faith in them. Keep watch on them from a distance, do not interfere unnecessarily. Intervene when required, preach when asked for, guide when they are faltering — this is the key to good parenting.

TIP OF THE DAY

If something bad happens, think of four steps to turn it into something good.
Suppose Your maid did not come today! Here are the four steps to make you feel good.
Doing housework will give you the required exercise.
You can take your afternoon nap peacefully without having to wait for her arrival.
You can clean all the cobwebs today which you have been putting off.
You are your own master, you can do the work as and when you feel like.

The Pawns

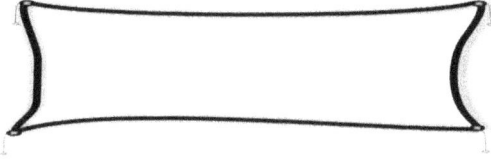

*C*hildren can be your best companions. They can be your source of joy. They can be your pride. But never turn them into your pawns. Life is not a game of chess. You cannot always make calculated moves. If you try to do so then life loses its charm and you lose the love and respect of others.

Athira was blessed with a son and daughter. The son was about eight years old and the daughter was two years old. Athira never had a good relationship with her in-laws. Though they lived in the same house, Athira lived on the first floor and her in-laws stayed on the ground floor. Athira was always suspicious of her in-laws. She would keep on spying on them, as to what they were doing, where were they going, what were they giving to their daughter and so on. Earlier, she used to ask all these things from her husband. When he got tired of answering these questions, she started asking the maidservant who also worked for her in-laws. The maid was a big gossipmonger. She would exaggerate things and tell Athira in a spicy manner. Somehow her mother-in-law got the wind of this. So she removed the maid. Now Athira had no other way of finding out as to what her in-laws are up to. This time, she thought of a new pawn in the form of her own son. She would coax her son to spend more time with the grandparents and when he came back home, she would ask him each and every detail. As the son grew up, he understood the subtle ways of his mother. He was genuinely fond of his grandparents. So he started spending more time with them. Now Athira was all the more worried. She felt that her in-laws had taken her son away from her. Her husband who was a silent spectator till now, opened his mouth and lashed his wife rudely for her wrong behaviour. Athira was aghast. It was the maze of her own creation from which she could not find an escape route.

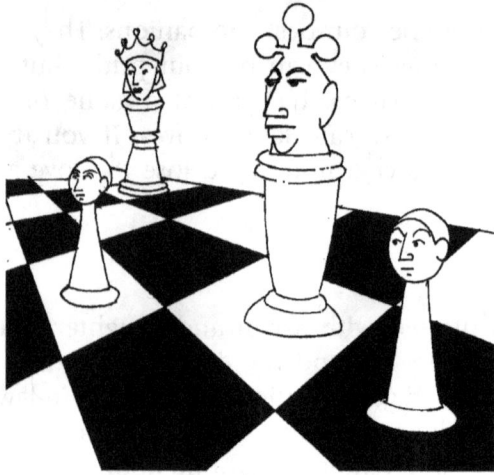

Some daughter-in-laws make the mistake of turning their children into pawns in their ongoing battles with their in-laws. This is wrong for it is not only foolish on your part, but it can also be harmful for the children. Children can serve as an ideal bridge between you and your in-laws because you both love them equally. Children may even help to keep channels of communication open during a cold war but using them as pawns to get information about their activities is a strict, 'no'. Instead, encourage your children to be close to their grandparents in good faith. There is a lot they can learn from their grandparents, which they will not find in text books or which you may not be able to teach them for want of time and patience. Values such as caring, sharing and giving are best taught by the grandparents for they have at their command a wealth of wisdom distilled from experience.

Remember, your in-laws are not your enemies. They are not out to snatch your children away. If your children love their grandparents, it does not mean they love you any less. So stop glaring at your in-laws, when they hug your children or buy special gifts for them. They are not out to bribe the children and steal their affection. They are merely conveying their affection towards them.

Grandparents can be a big support when it comes to raising your children. In today's hectic life, who has the time to sit with the children playing umpteen games, or telling them fairy tales or listening to the events of their day at school or feeding them patiently, spoon after spoon with love and affection. Only a grandparent can give such care.

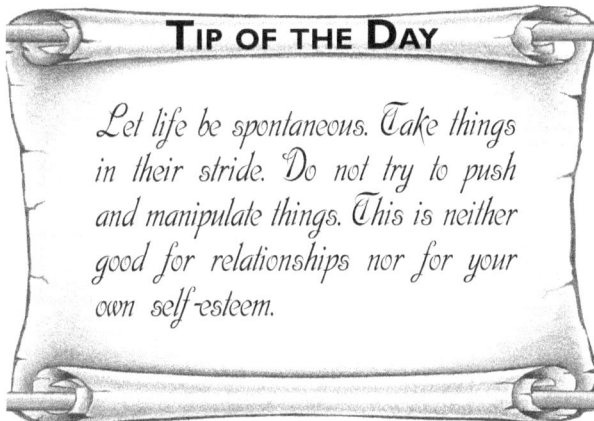

TIP OF THE DAY

Let life be spontaneous. Take things in their stride. Do not try to push and manipulate things. This is neither good for relationships nor for your own self-esteem.

It's My Life

Akbar once asked Birbal from where he had acquired all his wisdom.

Birbal said, "From fools. I observe their actions and try not to repeat their mistakes. In this way, I get wiser. There are enough fools around to provide anyone with wisdom. You just need to be observant."

♦ Learning from mistakes and experiences of others is the most effi cient and inexpensive way of learning.

♦ You can be to others only what you are to yourself. If you are honest with yourself, you will be honest with others as well.

♦ The more you will resist sufferings and miseries in life, the more they will trouble you.

The more you accept them, the more easily they will leave you.

Failing Health

We humans began our life form as a body and we still are primarily, a physical being. Without this body, we are nowhere. Health is a prime reason for stress. That is why, taking care of our body is important to us. With age, many problems crop up which not only hurt us physically but emotionally also. If we do not take care of our body, we can never be free of the ill effects of negative stress that always keeps affecting us. We may console ourselves that we are fit at the emotional or spiritual level, but it is a false sense of well being.

Meena was a fussy eater. She would eat very little to keep her figure slim and trim. Instead of eating healthy, she believed in crash diets. Whenever she felt the urge she would binge on junk foods and then shed the weight by crash diets. She never liked fruits, salads and other healthy foods. This made her most vulnerable to diseases. The trend continued even after she got married. Quite often, she would fall sick and would take days to recover. Since she was young, the body managed and she sailed through the early years of marital life. When her twin sons were born, the toll showed on her health. However much her mother-in-law coaxed her into eating nutritious diet, Meena just wouldn't touch it. She was afraid of putting on weight, so she started eating very less so as to shed the pregnancy weight as soon as possible. One day, she was bathing her four-month old son when she felt giddy and the baby slipped from her hands. His head hit the edge of the bathtub and started bleeding. Meena too fainted near him. The baby's howls alerted Meena's mother-in-law and she came rushing into the bathroom. Her timely intervention averted the crisis otherwise this minor fall would have turned into a major catastrophe for both the mother and the son. Meena got a good scolding from everyone including her husband. Now, she realized the value of good health.

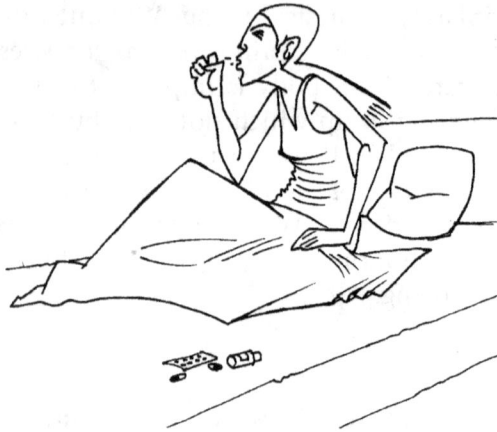

Since you are the pivotal point of your household, you cannot afford ill health. Your suffering passes on to other members of the family. So keep yourself mentally as well as physically fi t for the sake of everyone around you. Efforts to remain healthy not only keep you fi t, but also break the vicious circle of stress. For this, you may have to correct your lifestyle. There are three areas in your life which need attention to stay healthy — diet, exercise and relaxation.

Diseases such as migrains, hypertension, premenopausal blues, premenstrual stress (PMS) etc., may trouble you if you are under stress for a longer period of time. This stress increases the intensity of these problems, resulting in more stress. This turns into a vicious circle which becomes diffi cult to break. No medicine can help you. Doing meditation, keeping check on your emotions and not feeling stressed can help you.

It is said that *you are what you eat.* So eat a balanced and nutritious diet. Excessive consumption of any one type of food is not good. If you are obese then try to reduce weight safely. Start exercise regularly but the extent and pattern of exercise depends upon the age and physical condition of your body. If you do not feel inclined towards exercise, then the best and natural form of exercise is walking.

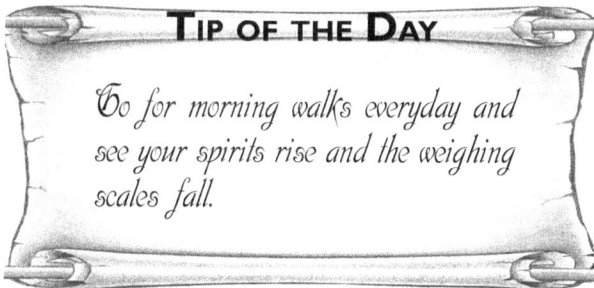

TIP OF THE DAY

Go for morning walks everyday and see your spirits rise and the weighing scales fall.

Be a Diya

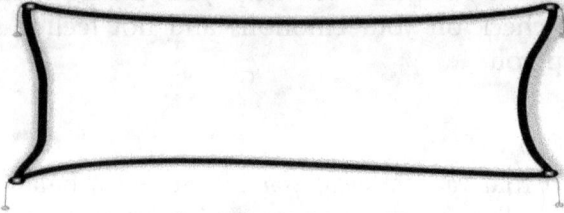

Family life has its own share of ups and downs, domestic dramas, personality clashes and what not. Don't you remember having arguments with your own parents, brothers and sisters before you got married? So what is the big deal or earth shattering if you ever had arguments with your in-laws or your husband? Do you blow your top at the slightest bit of friction? if you do, then you should better stop this matchstick behaviour and learn to keep your head cool instead of losing it at the slightest provocation.

Vinita married into a joint family. Her two sisters-in-law were unmarried at the time of her marriage. Vinita always had a hot temper. She could be easily provoked. She would argue over the matter and if not given due importance, she would shout on top of her voice. This kind of behaviour was not accepted at her in-laws, place. Being new to the place, at fi rst, she tried to suppress her anger. But old habits die hard. Soon, she came back to her normal self and started arguing with her in-laws over slightest pretext. But it was different here. Her in-laws' family was soft spoken and they rarely shouted at each other. So her shouting, raving and ranting was a new experience for them altogether. The mother-in-law tried to make her see reason. But Vinita's good sense was taken up by her anger. Now, her husband was asked to intervene. Each time he tried to pacify her, he saw no effect of his preachings. He stopped talking to her. The day arrived, when her in-laws called her parents and asked them to take her back. They told them in clear words to send her back only after she had learned to control her temper.

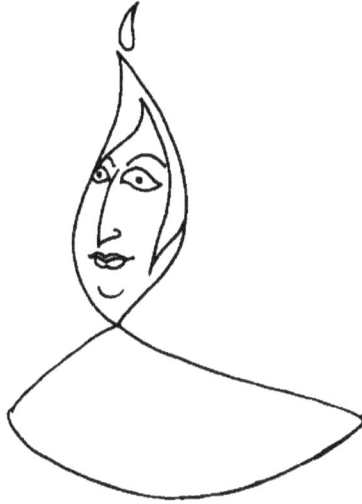

Getting angry at the slightest pretext can give rise to many stress related problems. We are not saying that you suppress your anger each time you feel angry. But you must learn to control your emotions and not get angry over little things. Instead of suppressing anger, control your temper. This will help you in maintaining good relations also.

Mental and physical problems make us weak and vulnerable. You may try to console yourself by keeping a brave front. You may be under the impression that you are free of stress. But what actually happens is that the negative effects of stress may be silently damaging your health, without your knowing this till you perceive the visible symptoms. By then, much damage has already been done. Remember, only a healthy body can continue to fi ght.

Relaxation is equally important although it does not mean merely resting. It means giving your mind a brief period of thoughtlessness. This is also known as meditation. So train your body and mind to relax.

TIP OF THE DAY

Become a diya - instead of being a matchstick, become a diya, which burns quietly, slowly and steadily till the last drop of oil. Do not react violently on impulse like a matchstick, learn to be patient like a diya.

Managing Home

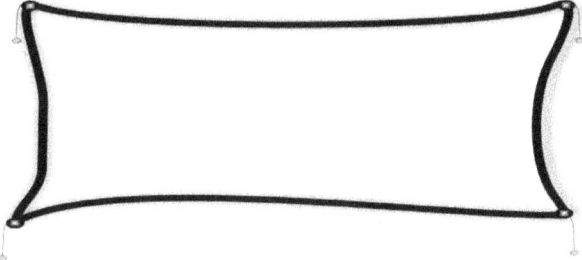

Your home is your pride. A housewife looks after her home and takes pride in it. Managing home is not an easy job. It is a full time job with no incentives or benefits of the job.

Geeta was brought up by *ayahs* since her mother was a working woman. Geeta, by choice, chose to be a housewife. But she always felt than an *ayah* is essential for bringing up a baby. When Geeta's daughter was born, she employed an *ayah* to look after the baby. But Geeta did not like the way that *ayah* handled her baby, so she fired her and started searching for another one. The next one handled the baby too roughly, so she was also fired. Geeta could not find a good one even after employing at least five or six *ayahs*. They all seemed dry, pathetic and rude. This started giving her stress because she could not entrust her precious child to someone who was not caring and affectionate. Geeta herself could have looked after the baby, had decided to put in some effort. A mother's care is definitely better than a hired help. But what came in the way was that Geeta had a vast social circle. She could not afford to be seen changing the baby's nappy or holding the baby in her arms and attending parties. Even though Geeta was a new mother, her mind was occupied most of the time by the thoughts of searching for a good servant or *ayah* rather than looking after her daughter.

Managing servants, these days is not an easy job. You have to be skilled in getting the work done by servants. They may try to take you for a ride. So be careful. Always keep good reliable servants. Pick them up from good organizations and have their credentials checked by the police. Do not treat servants shabbily. Do not try to extract work from them like a maniac. Remember, they are also human beings. So have patience and deal with them with care. Being a housewife, you should be profi cient enough in housework. Depending totally on the servants will make you a puppet in their hands. You must treat them as your helper and not as the ones who run your household. In this way, you will not feel depressed even if your servant goes away.

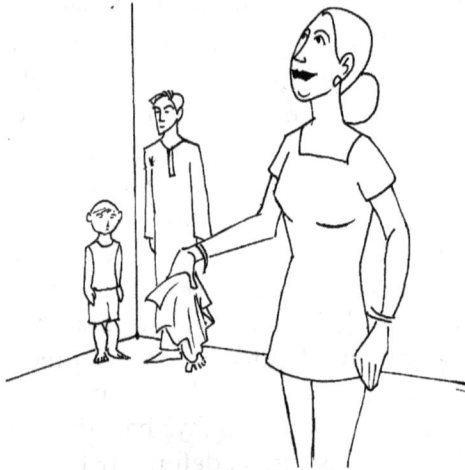

Home and hearth is your fort. Why get stressed over trivial things like servants or *ayahs*? Home management comes from experience. Intuition plays an important role in managing home. It is a blessing that you can devote all your time to your favourite place, i.e., your home. Just think of all those working women who balance their work and home perfectly. You are certainly in a better position than them because you have all the time in the world to shape your home as per your dreams. So why fret over it? Take advantage of this fact and manage your home without any stress.

Your child is the pivotal point of your total being. Why should you feel ashamed to look after your own baby? Do so with love, care and an open mind and find all your inhibitions melting away in that sweet toothless smile.

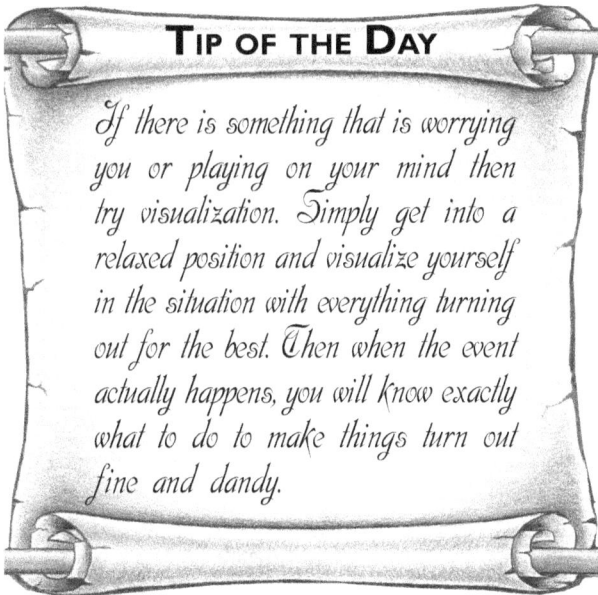

TIP OF THE DAY

If there is something that is worrying you or playing on your mind then try visualization. Simply get into a relaxed position and visualize yourself in the situation with everything turning out for the best. Then when the event actually happens, you will know exactly what to do to make things turn out fine and dandy.

Altered Feelings

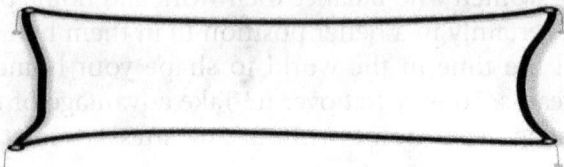

The extramarital affair can take birth within a family. In such situations, no one can guess what is going on under their nose. Your blind faith in your relations may cheat you at any point of time. So be careful when you place all your trust on people. You must learn to trust people but blind trust may hurt you. Both parties involved in an affair suffer in the end. So it's better to avoid such close shaves.

The most likely place for an affair to fl ourish outside home is the workplace, where people work in close proximity. Since you are a housewife, there is less chance of you being involved in an affair outside the home, but there are chances of your getting involved in an affair within the family but these are remote possibilities.

Deepti's husband was in Merchant Navy. He would be away from home for 3-4 months together. Deepti missed him badly but there was nothing she could do. In the absence of her husband, unknowingly, Deepti felt attracted towards her younger brother-in-law who was a cheerful person. No one objected to their going out together. Their chatting and laughing together was taken in good faith. Deepti also treated him like a good friend till one day, when he held her hand during a romantic movie, they were watching on television. One thing led to another. It was not before long everyone started suspecting them. Though the fear of losing her respect and position in the house and having to face her husband's wrath on his return terrifi ed Deepti, but she could not give up this relationship because he seemed to be her emotional anchor when her husband was away. But the tension was so much that it stole all the happiness away from her heart.

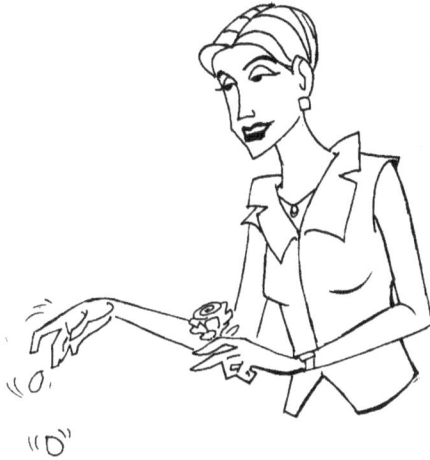

Your tension over an extramarital affair is quite justifi ed. This time, you are wrong. Whatever the initiating factor may be, cheating on your husband will not be acceptable by anyone, not even by your own conscience, that is why, it will prick you. You should stop such an affair immediately, before it's too late and go back to your life of bliss. Tell your husband, how lonely you feel without him. Maybe he can manage something.

Keep yourself occupied. Getting into an alleged relationship and then having to bear its repercussion throughout your life, is not the right way to deal with stress. Join some kitty parties, enroll into some hobby classes so that you do not have much free time on your hands. If you are qualifi ed, you may take up a job, part time or full time – as it suits you.

Get the gloom out of your mind. Remember, every dark cloud has a silver lining. That gleam will soon return to your life. You have to bide your time.

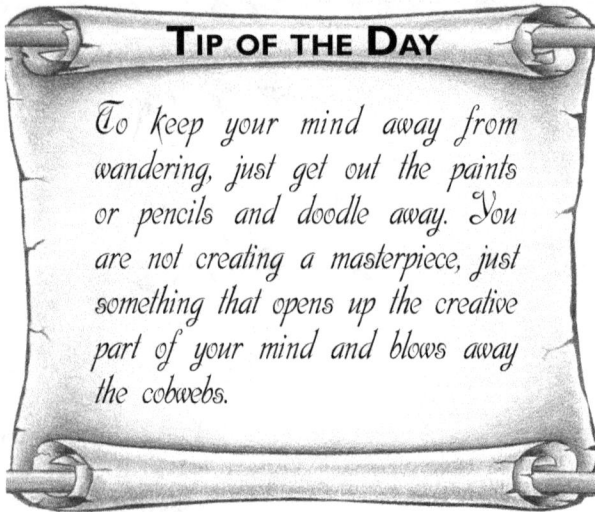

TIP OF THE DAY

To keep your mind away from wandering, just get out the paints or pencils and doodle away. You are not creating a masterpiece, just something that opens up the creative part of your mind and blows away the cobwebs.

Duty Bound

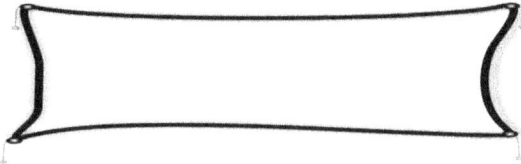

In most families, it is the duty of the son and his wife to look after the ageing parents. The daughters are absolved of all such duties once they get married. Such is our social system and is mostly acceptable to all. But what would a girl do who is emotionally attached to her parents and would like to do something for them? She keeps on thinking about their condition. Unable to do anything, she feels stressed and helpless.

Anjana's parents were weak and old. They stayed with her brother. Anjana's sister-in-law, Manu was always at loggerheads with them. Once when Anjana went to visit her parents, she found her mother slogging in the kitchen in sweltering heat while Manu sat in her air conditioned bedroom. Seeing Anjana unexpectedly, Manu came out of her room and tried to cover up the matter but damage was already done. Anjana accused her of not looking after her parents. Hearing this, Manu counter attacked and told her to set things right in her own house first because Anjana lived separately from her in-laws. In no time, a small matter flared into a big fight. Anjana had major arguments with her brother, and it turned out to be worse than anyone could have imagined. The two stopped talking to each other and from then on, whenever Anjana visited her parents, she would encounter with the gruff faces of her brother and sister-in-law. Later, she came to know that after her departure, they would take out their anger on the poor parents. Now Anjana regretted having acted so harshly. May be if she tried to make them see reason with a cool head, they would have understood and her relations with them would not have been spoiled. Now she has been alienated from the family and has no say in the family matters at all.

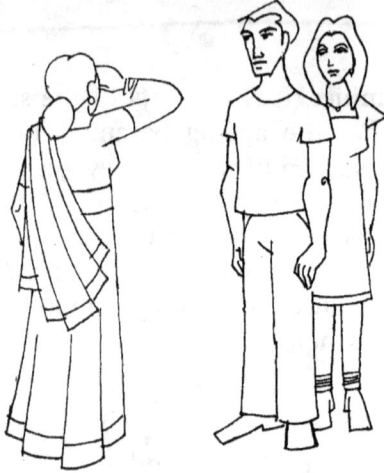

If your brother and his wife's behaviour is not good with your parents then it is a cause for concern. If they are ill treating your parents, then it is your right to intervene for the sake of your old parents. Be a passive watcher so long as you can manage. If you find the situation going out of hand, then only you should interfere. But try not to be too harsh on your brother and his family. You should not impose your ideas on them. In the long run, it is this relationship which will be your strength. So try to reach an amicable solution. Do not get depressed over your brother's behaviour if he does not accept your interference too kindly. To maintain your place and respect in your maternal home, do not get too involved in their daily matters. Speak only when you find the situation going out of hand.

If you can manage, bring your old parents with you, even if it is for a while. Once you are sure of your own feelings and your own family conditions, then you can suggest bringing the parents to your home forever. But if your own family conditions are not favourable, then do not press the matters too far. Help them quitely as much as you can.

Don't shy away from your duties as a daughter and place all the burden on you brother's shoulders. If you feel he is faltering away from his duties, then show him the right path by soft, comforting words. You are also married so put yourself into his position and imagine how would you feel if your sister-in-law talked to you in this manner about her parents and made you feel guilty? Remember, we are all riding in the same boat, so fights and accusations won't take us anywhere. If you expect your brother to be a *Shravan Kumar* then you should allow your husband also to act as *Shravan Kumar*.

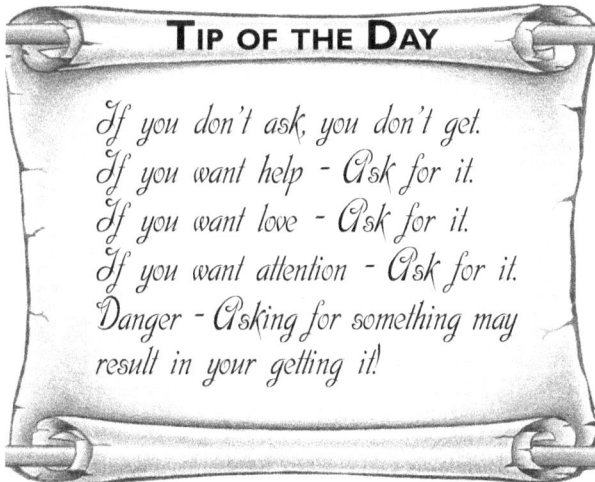

TIP OF THE DAY

If you don't ask, you don't get.
If you want help - Ask for it.
If you want love - Ask for it.
If you want attention - Ask for it.
Danger - Asking for something may result in your getting it!

Count Your Blessings

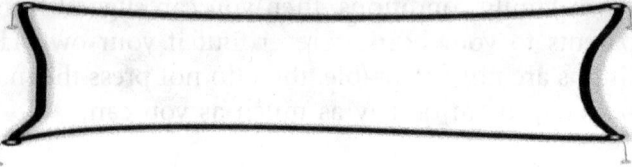

We often give more importance to others' opinion rather than concentrating on building our own character. We cannot stand rejection from others. Fear of others' opinion poses to be the greatest threat to us. This, in fact, is our own creation. By trying to impress others and thereby getting joy, you are indirectly giving the key of your own happiness in the hands of other people. If they want, they can make you happy, and if they want, they can make your life miserable.

Suruchi always gave more importance to others' opinion. When she got married, she was a bubbly young girl, but then she realised that her in-laws and others in the house did not want her to be so chirpy. So, she kept quiet. The house which came alive due to her lively chatter, became dull and quiet. When her husband went to Mumbai on deputation for two years, she stayed back wondering what would her in-laws say, if she expressed her desire to go with him. When her first daughter was born, there were mixed feelings in the family. Two years later, though Suruchi did not want another child yet she gave birth to one, fearing that people will call her an unlucky daughter-in-law who could not give an heir to the family. When her second daughter was born, there was clear downfall in mood in the house. Instead of rejoicing, it was more like mourning in the house. Suruchi was stressed, "What will people say now?" She cried inconsolably. Even though her husband tried to reason with her that it made no difference to him whether he had two sons or two daughters, nothing seemed to penetrate Suruchi, who was perturbed over what people will say. She was stressed over something on which she had no control.

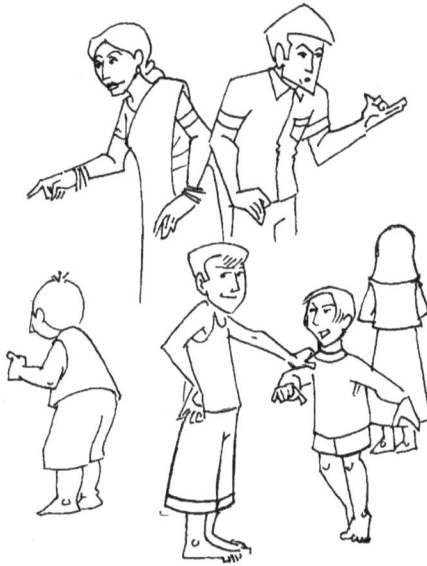

Why should you live your life on the guidelines issued by others? This happens when you cannot stand rejection. Fear of others' opinion is the greatest threat that you have created for yourself. By trying to impress others and thereby getting joy, you are simply becoming a puppet in the hands of others, who will make you dance to their tune. You are then reduced to a slave by mortgaging your happiness on the mercy of others. Your happiness and contentment should rest in your hands and not in somebody else's hands. You should do any work primarily from the point of view of your own satisfaction. You should derive joy from what you are doing. It should not wait for the time when somebody will come and appreciate your work.

Do not give undue importance to other people's views about you as to whether they know your calibre or capabilities or whether they overestimate or underestimate you. Even if you are not able to come up to everyone's expectations, it should not cause much concern. Everyone has different calibre and everyone is entitled to different opinion of his or herself and others. You cannot win them all. To have a desire to be at the top always and to seek appreciation from everyone is highly illusory and is bound to give you stress. So give up this feeling and lead a normal life, which shall bring you satisfaction and happiness.

Your joy should not wait for the time when somebody will come and appreciate your work. Your estimation in your own eyes should be much more important. Other people's comments should be taken only objectively as an opportunity to assess yourself and take only corrective measures, if required.

TIP OF THE DAY

Time to put up your feet for the day and enjoy. When the entire family sleeps till noon on holidays, why should you wake up early and slog in the kitchen scurrying up a princely breakfast for them? Select such a menu for the day, which only needs heating and ready to serve. Now relax and have a refreshing sleep.

Relationships

One day when Akbar and Birbal were out hunting, the emperor pointed to a crooked tree and asked, "Why is that tree crooked?"

Birbal answered, "That tree is crooked because it is the son-in-law of all the trees in the forest."

"Why do you say that," asked Akbar.

Birbal quoted a proverb, "A dog's tail and a son-in-law are always crooked"

Akbar retorted, "Is my son-in-law also crooked?"

"Of course, Your Majesty, if we go according to the saying", replied Birbal.

"Then have him crucified", ordered Akbar.

A few days later, Birbal had three crosses made — one of gold, one of silver and one of copper.

Akbar asked, "What are these for?"

"Your Majesty, one of them is for you, one for me and one for Your Majesty's son-in-law."

"But why are we to be crucified?" asked Akbar.

"Because" replied Birbal, "we are all sons-in-laws of someone."

Akbar laughed and said, "Well then, let my son-in-law go."

The dialogue between Akbar and Birbal teaches us a simple truth. We are all related to each other. Relationships are a part of our lives. Since we cannot change the people, the best thing, we can do is change our attitude. Sometimes, you can change your 'wavelength' to suit the other person. Such changes are not compromise, it is wisdom. And the wise are ready to do anything to maintain a more profi table, congenial relationship.

There are different roles a woman plays during a lifetime. She is a daughter, sister, a caring wife, daughter-in-law, mother and ultimately, a mother-in-law. A caring attitude and endurance go a long way.

With a sweet tongue and kindness,

You can drag an elephant by the hair.

An Obedient Daughter

They gave you birth and nurtured you till you were old enough to fl y away from their nest. But it is not easy for us humans to break away the loving ties so easily as birds do. We remain attached to our parents throughout our lives and are always there for each other through thick and thin.

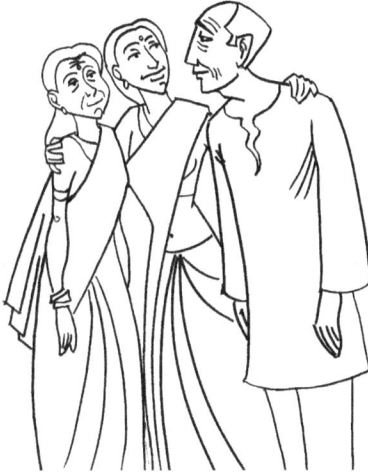

If you parents are old and disabled, then it is a cause for concern. If they have someone to look after them then it is good, otherwise it is certainly the girl's duty to look after her old parents. There are so many people in our society today who live with their daughters because they have no one else to look after them. This eases up tension and worry over their well being for the daughter as well as for them.

If you parents are fi nancially weak, then the daughter feels like walking on a tight rope. She has to take her husband's permission before helping her old parents fi nancially. If she is fi nancially independent, then she need not take anyone's permission. But a nod from her husband is required, if she is a housewife.

Do you take permission from your husband for each and every thing? Does he seek your permission while bringing his parents to his house? Certainly not. Then why do you think you should take his permission in looking after your parents? Yes, you may seek his advice on how to settle these matters. You may apprise him of the situation and seek his opinion. Leaving him totally unaware will certainly give rise to tension at home and strain your relationship.

Leading a lonely life is the biggest curse, especially in old age. If your parents are old and leading a lonely life, then it is a cause enough for worry. Try to bring them to your house so that you can tend to them. After all, they are your parents who looked after you all your life. Don't get stressed over things like what will people say and so on.

You love your parents and want the best for them. So there is bound to be stress if you fi nd them in a diffi cult situation. But you need to manage that stress because action is what is needed in such situations not brooding in a corner.

I know of a family that had two daughters and a son. All the children were married and settled. The parents lived with the son but the son and his wife did not look after them well. Seeing this, the two sisters got together. One of the sisters was working while the other was a housewife. They talked the matter over with their brother and came to a solution. The sister who was not working rented an apartment near her house. The parents shifted into that house. The father used to get some pension. The son was asked to pay for the rent. The daughters arranged for the groceries and other things and father used his pension for

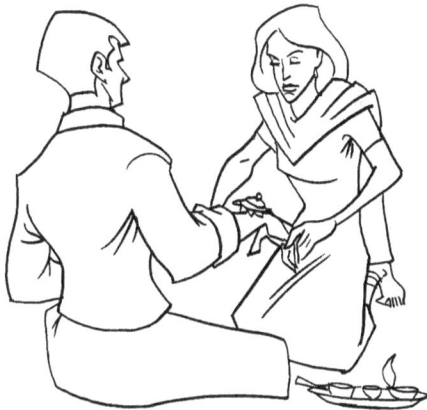

their personal expenses. The arrangement suited everyone. The parents also enjoyed their independence and felt more relaxed. Each family visited them on alternate Sundays. Life was easier for everyone now. In this way, everyone shared the burden and parents even managed to save some money from their pension which was later distributed equally among the three children when both the parents died.

An Understanding Sister

You spent your childhood with your brother. You must have had your share of happy moments as well as fighting spells. But that does not lessen your love for each other. Being almost of the same age as your brother, you can understand his views, ideas and feelings easily and respond to them in a positive manner. You two can be a pillar of support for each other throughout life. So nurture this relationship with love and care. It will reap great benefits.

Once your brother gets married, a new responsibility is added to his life, which is not only dear to his heart, it also keeps growing with passing years. You may not approve of his wife, but since, he has married her, she is as much a part of your family, as you yourself are. So accept her with open arms. Do not be prejudiced in dealing with her. Teach her the rules of your house and never ridicule her in front of anyone.

This is one relation which is dear to every woman's heart, no matter what. You may be at loggerheads with your sister-in-law, you may be angry with your brother for not giving enough time to the parents, but when it comes to his children, you melt like butter. Maybe you see the replica of your brother in them, who was once as innocent and helpless as his children are now. This brings in a surge of fresh sisterly love and you start doting on them.

Now that you are grown up, you may be each other's best friends. So stop bullying each other and understand the other person's point of view. You must appreciate the fact, that each of you have your individual life and the bond which binds you and your brother together is your parents. Based on that bond, your relationship should grow stronger each day. New relations will keep adding to it during the course of time. Make sure they strengthen your bond and not weaken it.

A Dutiful Daughter-in-Law

All relationships – with friends, neighbours, parents, brother, sister – need a lot of careful nurturing. So why not the relationship with in-laws? There is a drawback in this relationship. In-laws are in the unfortunate position of being not quite the same as family and are seldom considered friends. We neither feel the spontaneous love for them that we do for our blood relations or immediate family nor are we willing to give them the time and importance that we give to our friends.

Relations with in-laws have to be watered with plenty of care, patience and understanding. Invest time in your in- laws. It will bear rich dividends. In the bargain, you will not lose anything. Instead, it will make your stock with them soar. It is a guaranteed, time tested win-win deal. Each of us is someone's daughter-in-law, mother-in-law or sister-in-law. And since, we are neither wicked nor mean, there is no rule that defines that in-laws are necessarily bad.

Why, then is there such a fear of in-laws? Why are in-laws the butt of so much criticism? Fear of in-laws is like fear of *Tapka* (fear of the unknown). Their image has been ingrained in a young girl's mind in such a way that she views them as the villains in every domestic melodrama at homes. Films and serials on television have only added fi re to the fuel.

Go to any *Ladies' Sangeet* on the night before the wedding and you will hear women singing naughty songs criticising the girl's would be in-laws. But there are hardly any songs which glorify the in-laws.

In-laws are undoubtedly the cornerstone of all successful marriages. I am not saying that you must love your in-laws, I am simply trying to emphasize on the concept of co-existence. You must learn to co-exist happily with minimum tension. A good working relationship with the in-laws is important if you want to keep your family happy and well knit. Do not forget, it is these little things that go a long way in paving the path for the big and important things.

There are numerous jokes about in-laws. One of them goes like this – You may have seen a certain kind of cactus with long, sharp leaves. The leaves are green with yellow borders. The edges are sharp and thorny. This plant is called the **mother-in-law's tongue!**

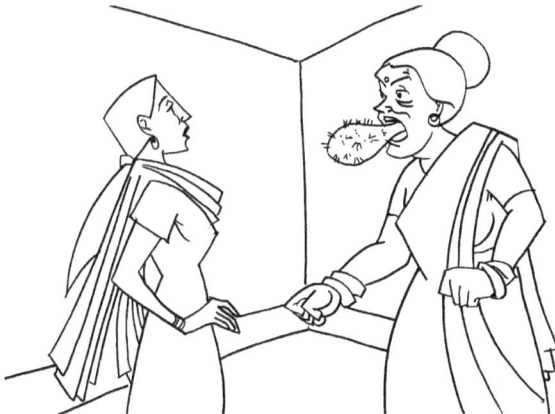

In the final analysis, deciding to be happy is as important as being happy. If you allow the constant squabbling to get you, you are bound to be stressful and unhappy. On the other hand, if you believe that happiness is a state of mind, smiles and laughter will come back into your life. So the next time, when you have a hot discussion with your mother-in-law over the maid or with your sister-in- law over whose turn it is to make the *chapatis* or you see your father-in-law poking his nose in front of your smart friends... be cool. It will make you realise that such petty issues are not worth staking your happiness for.

A Caring Wife

If you wish to have happiness for a lifetime, then learn to care for your better half. Because caring for your husband is what the twoway street called marriage is all about. The love and respect of your better half with whom you may spend 40 or 50 springs is far more important than any diamond necklace, you would preserve for similar number of years.

A perfect couple is like a perfect apple — diffi cult to fi nd. Maybe, you have come across one that looked perfect, but you couldn't tell what it would really be like unless you cut it. It may be rotten inside.

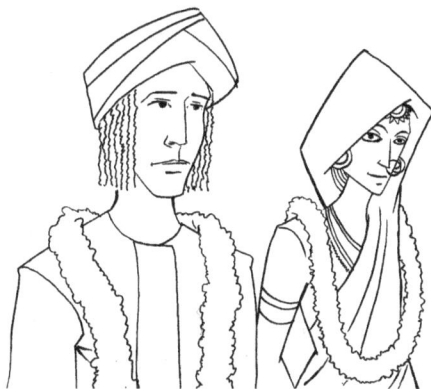

Please do not get me wrong. I am simply saying that you can never get a perfect couple. Use your mental knife to cut out your husband's bad points and you will fi nd him too good to be true. Fortunately, God has blessed us with a memory which can be as sharp as a razor and when need be, it can be as bad as an erased fl oppy. In fact, it can be erased at will and only what you want to remember can remain in it.

Try it out. This can lead to happiness in your married life.

Pygmalion was a character in Greek mythology who believed so strongly in the beauty of the statue he had carved that it came to life. So the fi rst step towards a good relationship with your husband is having confi dence in him. Your opinion of your husband infl uences his behaviour and improves his confi dence. You can have a better half who is ten feet tall or ten inches tall. The choice is yours.

You must realise that to be happy, you must ensure that your husband is a happy person. Very little is needed to make your husband feel great. It costs almost nothing. You do not have to gift a designer wrist watch or an expensive tie to make him happy. Just a smile, a wink, a kiss – anyone or all of them in any order – and that's about it. He will feel on the top of the world. You do not even have to do it everyday. Once in a while, will do the trick. Try it!

One thing sure, you cannot change him. So it is best to accept him as he is. If you still want to try changing a few of his habits which you disapprove – like his stinking socks, wet towel on the bed, papers scattered all over the study, dirty dishes piled up on the table, his shaving kit spread all over the dressing table, then have patience, give him time to understand why you do not like these things and then do it gently over a few years while making some compromises for your own behaviour too which is not acceptable to him. It is not tit for tat, I would call it give and take.

Always remember that your better half is unique so treat him as such. Think of all the little things you can do for your better half. Thoughtful gestures can make your partner feel loved and cared for.

As a parent, your moment of triumph is when your children grow up to be fi ne human beings. It does not happen overnight. There is a lot of hard work and care which goes in churning out these best specimens which stole your heart when you fi rst held them in your arms, years ago.

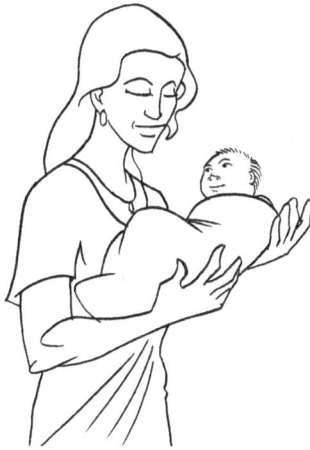

Managing children, since times immemorial has always been a tough job. The challenge lies in making the tough job as simple as possible. Raising children is purely an art which you can hope to master with practice and patience. If they are nurtured and encouraged and given the right kind of atmosphere to grow they prove to be our assets but if not, they are likely to become liabilities. So, to be able to manage the children, we must first learn to manage ourselves.

Parents are the anchors for their children. They watch you and learn a lot from your behaviour. So let us do what we would like them to do when they grow up. Share with them what you read, write or think. Respect your elders so that they do the same when the time arrives. Remember, they are watching us as God is watching us from heaven. Do not worry if you cannot provide your child with a chauffeur driven car, or you cannot treat them to the best of restaurants. There is something more precious than all these material things which you can offer them — your love. Be there to comfort them when they get hurt or when they are feeling low. Make sure that they get the best smiles life can offer and always be there to hold them, if they stumble. When they have tears in their eyes, they should have the confidence that their mother will be there to wipe them away. This confidence will stay with them all their lives leading to a bond beyond this world.

Be a friend

Give them this confidence that whenever they need, you are there to help them. Never mock them or laugh at their silly doubts or belittle their stupid thoughts. Give them the confidence to confide everything in you. Earning your child's confidence is the biggest lottery you would ever win in life.

Spare a moment

Spend time with your kids. Play games, read books, help with their homework and enquire about their friends. Let them open their hearts to you.

Never criticize them

Shouting at or beating them or criticizing them in front of others makes the children feel small, confused and hurt and they become more stubborn by receding into their shell.

Step into their shoes

Do not compare your children's situation with your own which existed a quarter of a century ago when you were their age. Things change, so should you. Put yourself in their shoes and understand that your children have feelings and needs which are different from yours.

Do not preach but teach them

Your role as a parent is incomplete unless you take pain to teach your children some essential coping skills. Remember to help them walk these five steps to make them turn into better human beings.

- ♦ Teach them to be responsible.
- ♦ Teach them to learn to lose and to enjoy winning.
- ♦ Give them the best education within your means.
- ♦ Expose them to various situations and let them grow independently.
- ♦ Stimulate their creativity.

Relaxation Techniques

Relaxation techniques are useful in preventing stress and lowering your physical signs of stress. Keep aside fifteen minutes in your day to relax and you will feel rejuvenated throughout.

Before we begin with the relaxation techniques, let us learn about the six events schedule as stress buster. You may take a close look at your daily routine and choose up to six events that regularly recur. These events can be from boiling the milk in the morning to cutting vegetables in the afternoon. Just like you watch your favourite television soap while cutting vegetables, similarly, add on any of the relaxation technique which can easily blend with your activity and practice it for a fixed period. The period should be decided by you. It should be such that you can easily accommodate.

Let's take the example of cutting vegetables. Suppose you do it before your kids come back from school. Till now, you have preferred watching your favourite soap on TV while cutting vegetables. That means you are already used to cutting vegetables unconsciously, while being engaged in another activity. For a housewife, this is an event which occurs everyday. Now instead of serfing on the TV, do the **Centering Breathing Exercise** for a fixed period while cutting vegetables everyday. This way, you ensure a continuous physical relaxation exercise regimen, each day.

The value of this approach lies in its painless

reprogramming. The new routine is slipped in alongside the old routine or it may be added to the existing, accepted sequence of events. By doing this, you defuse the negative impact of a change that you are inflicting upon yourself. As human nature, our body and our psyche oppose any sudden change in our lifestyle. But with this kind of approach, you do not feel this negative impact and start to feel the benefits immediately.

Try and do this harmless exercise. You will find this experience exhilirating. The positively altered states of the body and mind even for brief periods throughout your day will prevent the otherwise unmitigated buildup of stress. In this way, you counteract the stress as it comes. Now you will not carry an ever increasing load on your shoulders.

Aerobic exercises require rapid movements of the body. They also help in releasing the bound up energy in tight muscles by utilizing this energy for movements. This provides immediate relaxation to the body and mind. Aerobics also stimulate the release of endorphins (body's natural pain killers) in the body which gives a pleasant feeling to the mind.

- ♦ The first and foremost step is put on music with beats.
- ♦ Move your body along the beats.
- ♦ A fast music track will ensure rapid movement of the body.
- ♦ Try stretching each part of the body on the beats of the music.
- ♦ Soon, you will find your body feeling relaxed.

Have you ever put a baby to sleep? A crying baby becomes quiet the moment you start rocking him in your arms. He relaxes and slowly goes off to sleep. Get into a rocking chair and rock to and fro and fi nd your tension vanish. Similarly, swinging on a swing (*jhoola*) also reduces tension. These activities produce a sensation of lightness and create a feeling of mental euphoria which relaxes the body and mind.

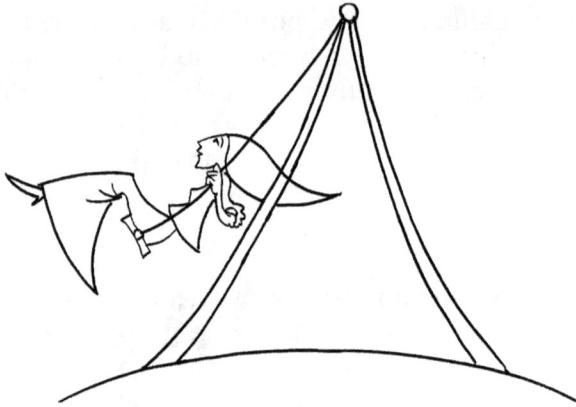

After a hectic physical activity, it is very important to relax your body.

The best position to experience true relaxation is by lying on your back. First of all, the heart no longer need to pump uphill to the brain, secondly, it need not maintain adequate pressure to ensure the return of venous blood from the legs. So your blood pressure is quickly reduced or in other words, normalized.

♦ Lie on your back in a comfortable, quiet room.

- ♦ Separate your feet to about shoulder width and allow them to fall outwards.
- ♦ Turn the palms of your hands upwards so that the back of your hands are in contact with the fl ow. This is important as your fi ngers are richly supplied with nerves and pressure receptors that constantly relay information to your brain. When the hands are turned upwards, this fl ow of information or stimulus is suspended.
- ♦ Stretch your arms at a considerable distance from your sides.
- ♦ Check that your head and body are in a straight line.
- ♦ Close your eyes.
- ♦ Begin with concentrating on your breathing.
- ♦ Slowly inhale through your nose, expanding your adbomen before allowing the air to fi ll your lungs.
- ♦ Hold the breath till you feel comfortable, then exhale.
- ♦ Reverse the process as you exhale.
- ♦ Make tight fi sts, hold for fi ve seconds and relax. Do this three times.
- ♦ Pay attention to the different sensations of tension and relaxation in your body.
- ♦ Concentrate on the sensations. If your mind tends to wander, then bring it back on line with conscious effort.
- ♦ Repeat it with each part of the body feeling tension and relaxation of each muscle.

By stretching various muscles, the pockets of tension and tightness are released. The muscles get relaxed which were previously tight due to stress response. If done correctly, stretching can promote relaxation and reduce stress. Have you ever noticed a cat stretch herself? she does it with such perfection that by just watching it, we can feel released. So try this slow and deliberate body stretch.

Stand straight or sit up straight while doing stretching exercises.

- As you stretch think about a specifi c area. Imagine the tension leaving as you gently take this area into comfortable limit.

- Exhale into the stretch and inhale on the release.

- Breathe deeply and slowly continuously – do not hold your breath.

- For the backbone — Let your head move down to your chest and exhale. You will feel a gentle stretch on the back of the neck and shoulders.

- Roll your left ear towards your left shoulder while inhaling. Drop your chin to your chest again while exhaling.

- Repeat the same with your right ear.

- Drop the arms sideways and push both the shoulders forward.

- Slowly raise them towards your ears and circle them back and downwards to the starting point.

- After two or three rotations, you can change directions.

Shaking is akin to shivering when you feel cold. Shivering is body's natural attempt to produce warmth through vibration and movement. Shaking is the fastest and most effective form of relaxation. In shaking all over, this approach is amplified and applied, specifically and systematically to all the major joints of the body.

- ♦ You may begin shaking with your feet and ankles. Transfer all your weight onto your one leg and straighten the other leg slightly out of the side. Now make rapid movements with the straight leg, so that the foot moves very rapidly.

- ♦ Continue for about ten seconds. Then change legs and repeat.

- ♦ You may do the same process with knees and thighs, pelvis, buttocks and the lower back.

- ♦ Wrists, elbows and shoulders come next in the shaking process.

- ♦ While shaking the head and neck, keep your facial muscles relaxed and mouth partially open. Begin making small, rapid movements in the neck. Do not throw the head from side to side but set up a rapid vibration. By keeping the mouth open, your cheeks and lips can also participate in the movement.

- ♦ You may run the shaking process through your whole body as many times as you feel necessary emphasizing those areas that need extra attention.

- ♦ After a good shake, you will feel more relaxed and awake.

Meditation helps you calm the mind so that you can think straight in a relaxed state of mind. The goal is not for immediate relaxation, but to increase serenity. Meditation puts you in control of your thoughts which usually tend to run haywire. Most of the time, we are either thinking about the past or the future. Meditation forces us to be present in the moment and to observe our thought processes. Meditation will not reap its benefits unless you practise it on a regular basis. Also you need to devote sometime to learn this process because it is time consuming initially. Do not lose heart if you are not able to master this art in the first few sittings.

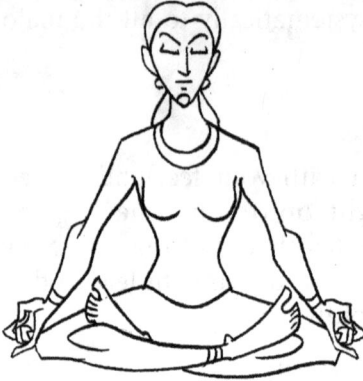

You may begin doing meditation for 10 to 15 minutes, once a day initially. Increase this to 20 minutes and then twice a day. Avoid meditating just before going to bed or you will be too energised to sleep. Though there are various techniques of meditation, you may choose whichever suits you the best.

♦ Choose a quiet room where you will not be interrupted for 15-20 minutes.
♦ Take time to relax, do not rush.
♦ When you feel thoroughly relaxed, concentrate on your breathing.

- Your breathing should be slow and even.
- Close your eyes now.
- Slowly breathe a rhythmic word (like *OM*) over and over again in your mind as you breathe in and out.
- Continue this for 10-15 minutes.
- To come back to the real world, chant the word aloud, deliberately and slowly.
- Pay special attention to your breathing.
- Be aware of your body and your posture.
- Open your eyes and look around.
- After a minute, stand up and stretch.

With practice, you will eventually reach the point when you will feel detached from your body and physical surroundings while meditating. The world will fade away from your awareness, you will be in touch with your innermost self. You will feel deeply relaxed and thoroughly energized.

When meditation is practised each day, its positive effects are many. Meditation does not provide an escape from the daily life but it prepares you for it. When you meditate, you attain silence and become calm. The silence and calm moments with oneself help the troubled mind and seek solution to the problem that has been lurking in the mind for so long.

Meditation is a process of self discovery. With very little time for ourselves, we tend to drift away from our inner self. Meditation helps us unite with our own self and provides a clear solution to our pressing psychological and related problems.

Essence of Spirituality

I ndian Philosophy propagates certain important things that we may call 'the essence of spirituality'.

❖

What is life? Our body spends a short time on earth – that is what is life. You may spend this time in happiness or in unhappiness. But you must understand that there is no points in spoiling this brief time by your own thinking and acts and remain unhappy and stressed throughout the short journey.

❖   —

Everyone is aware of the fact that one has to die, yet all of us want to believe that we are immortal. Everything in this world is temporary. We are not here for good. We tend to overestimate our problems as if they are permanent. We forget the fact that when life itself is temporary then nothing else can be permanent. So why trouble ourselves unduly for things that are of a short duration only?

❖

We feel that we are important enough for the situation to change itself to suit our requirements. We also feel that situations are important enough to feel happy or sad about. But situations keep changing. Change is the law of nature. So if everything is temporary, when nothing is really very important, then why worry too much?

❖

Everything is not in your hands. Everything is not because of you. Most of our problems arise because we attach too much importance to ourselves. We think that we are in charge of things and everything depends upon us. We get worried and anxious when we find that while we should be in charge of the situation, this is not actually so. In other words, we are psychologically not ready to accept our inadequacy and insignificance in the scheme of things. We feel, we will be able to change the situation. But when we are unable to do so, we get annoyed and it hurts our ego. We feel guilty about our own failures.

We have to free ourselves from this delusion and be prepared to face them. Then there will be no room for regret, disappointment or unhappiness.

Cherish Happiness

Happiness is the ultimate objective of human life. Happiness, as a concept is unique to human beings. Other living things have sensations of security, satisfaction, pleasure or enjoyment but happiness is something above these sensations which they never experience. We have all felt happy but if I ask you to define happiness, you will be at a loss of words.

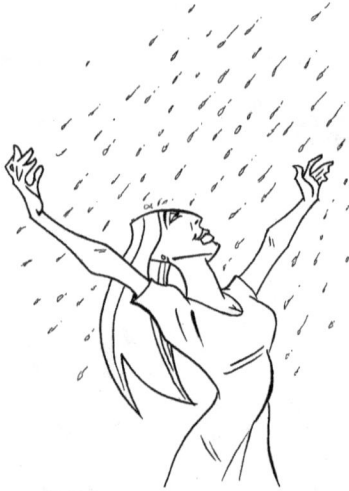

It is indeed very difficult to define happiness. You may say it is a feeling to be enjoyed, not described. Very true, but we can surely identify some of the key elements of what constitutes happiness.

♦ Happiness is associated with peace of mind.

172

- Happiness brings tranquillity.
- Happiness spreads to others.
- Happiness is not a momentary sensation. It is a longterm feeling.
- Happiness does not erode. It has an element of permanency.
- Happiness is self generated. It does not depend upon external factors.

To many of us, happiness seems to be something elusive. It is something that is not with us right now but might come to us sometime later in life. We have our set rules that if we achieve a particular thing, or if we reach a particular position, we will be happy. Happiness seems like a mysterious thing that is likely to come to us sometime in future, but is never a part of our today. It is like a milestone which we hope to pass one day.

1. **HUMILITY** — Be humble. Nothing brings peace of mind as surely as humility.
2. **SIMPLICITY** — Simplicity shows in your actions, behaviour and interaction with others.
3. **HONESTY** — Honesty is being truthful to your own self.
4. **GENEROSITY** — Generosity is about accepting mistakes and imperfections, whether they are of your own making or of others. Acceptance without argument or agitation is the first step towards generosity.
5. **FORGIVENESS** — Forgiving frees you of all negative feelings. So why carry the burden of revenge? Forgive and forget and live life stress free.

6. **BE EMPATHETIC** — Stepping in the other person's shoes and seeing the world from their point of view.

7. **BE CONSIDERATE** — Share your happiness.

8. **BE A LEARNER** — Learn from your mistakes.

9. **ADMIT MISTAKES** — Accept your fault and give yourself an opportunity to improve.

10. **SENSE OF SUPERIORITY** — Things are neither superior nor inferior in this world. Things are only different.

Live a stress free life and spread happiness all around you.

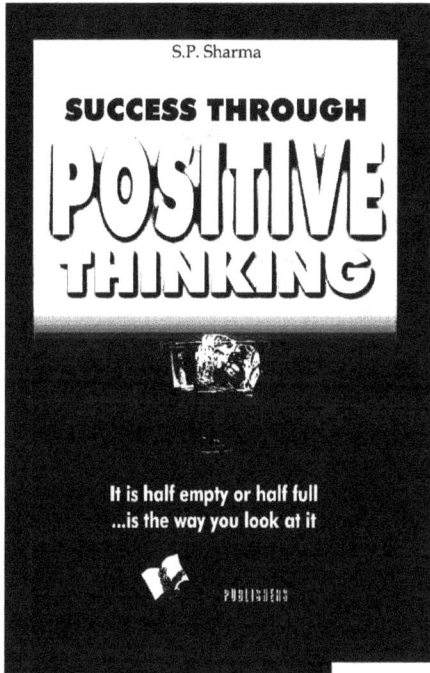

SUCCESS THROUGH
POSITIVE
THINKING

Author: S.P. Sharma
Format: Paperback
Language: English
Pages: 176
Price: ₹ 96
Publishers: V&S PUBLISHERS

PEACE
of MIND

Author: Hair Datt Sharma
Format: Paperback
Language: English
Pages: 174
Price: ₹ 96
Publishers: V&S PUBLISHERS

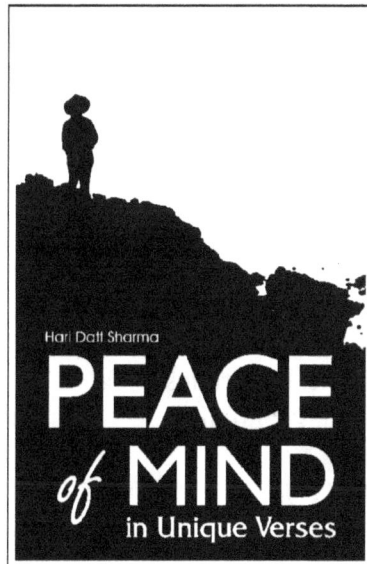

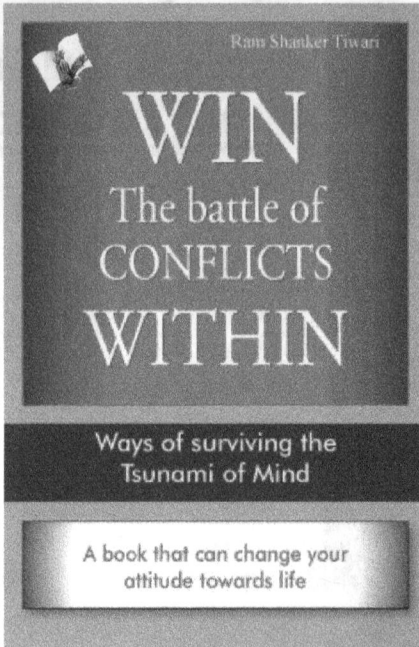

WIN
The battle of
CONFLICTS
WITHIN

Author: Dr. Ram Shanker
Format: Paperback
Language: English
Pages: 260
Price: ₹ 175
Publishers: V&S PUBLISHERS

Ram Shanker Tiwari

WIN
The battle of
CONFLICTS
WITHIN

Ways of surviving the
Tsunami of Mind

A book that can change your
attitude towards life

EXPLORE
YOUR
HIDDEN
TALENTS

Author: Hair Datt Sharma
Format: Paperback
Language: English
Pages: 174
Price: ₹ 96
Publishers: V&S PUBLISHERS

Dr. Aparna Chattopadhyay

EXPLORE
YOUR
HIDDEN
TALENTS

Over 40
self-analysis modules
to help you bring out your
hidden potential and
excel in career

V&S PUBLISHERS

www.ingramcontent.com/pod-product-compliance
Lightning Source LLC
Chambersburg PA
CBHW050523270326
41926CB00015B/3048